TOP FITNESS ADVICE

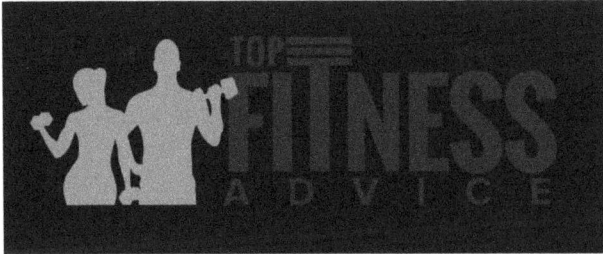

7-DAY WEIGHT LOSS

2nd Edition

Total Body Transformation –
Drop A Dress Size Fast With 7
Days of Recipes, Exercises, &
Healthy Habits!

LINDA WESTWOOD

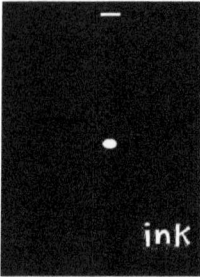

First published in 2015 by Venture Ink Publishing

Copyright © Top Fitness Advice 2019

All rights reserved.

For more information about the contents of this book or questions to the author, please contact Linda Westwood at linda@topfitnessadvice.com

Disclaimer

Table of Contents

Would you prefer to listen to my book, rather than read it?

Download the audiobook version for free!

If you go to the special link below and sign up to Audible as a new customer, you can get the audiobook version of my book completely free.

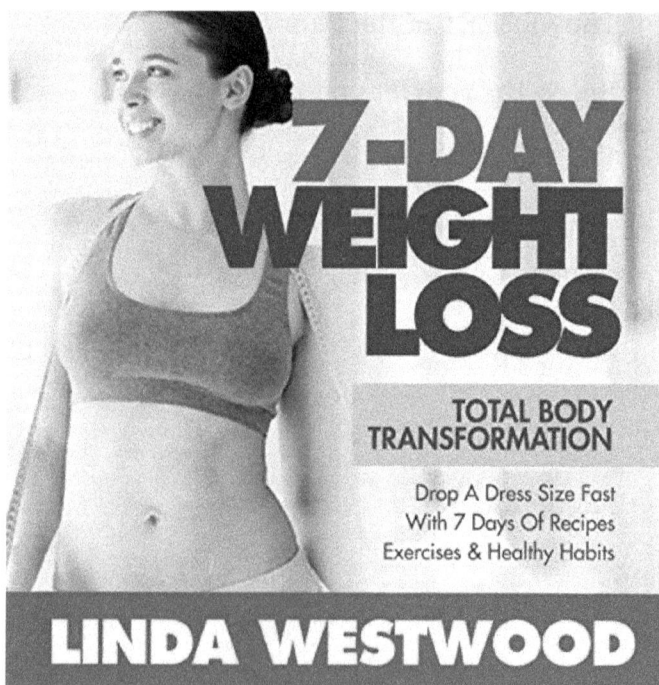

Go here to get your audiobook version for free:

TopFitnessAdvice.com/go/7day

Who is this book for?

Do you need a *strong* kick-start with your weight loss?

Do you need to lost weight *FAST*?

Do you have an event coming up that you need to *drop a dress size for?*

If you answered "Yes" to any of those questions – **this book is for you!**

I am going to share with you the most effective way to slim down and drop an entire dress size in just 7 days!

I have put it all together in this awesome Drop A Dress Size in 7 Day *rapid* weight loss plan!

The best part about is that you are going to see amazing results and this will *TRANSFORM YOUR BODY JUST 7 DAYS*!

You can be a complete beginner or someone who works out regularly, it doesn't matter!

If this sounds like it could help you, then keep reading...

What will this book teach you?

Inside, I will teach you one of the best ways to quickly lose weight, especially targeted to dropping an entire dress size within a week!

You will feel the healthiest you have ever felt – have the most energy you have ever had – and the fat will be melting *constantly!*

How?

Because you're going to be eating well, and doing some of the most effective workouts that accelerates body transformation in a short period of time.

In this book, I give you the plan right in front of you that will change your life – all you have to do is follow it!

One of the most important things for you to realize when reading this book is that this weight loss plan *really does work!*

However...

For you to achieve *real success*, you HAVE to apply this to your life.

This is where most people fail – they read through the entire book but do nothing. You MUST try your best to apply as you read through the book!

Discover Scientifically-Proven "Shortcuts" & "Hacks" to Lose Weight FASTER (With Very Little Effort)

For this month only, you can get Linda's best-selling & most popular book absolutely free – *Weight Loss Secrets You NEED to Know.*

Get Your FREE Copy Here:

TopFitnessAdvice.com/Bonus

Discover scientifically-proven tips to help you lose weight faster and easier than ever before. With this book, readers were able to improve their weight loss results and fitness levels. So, it's highly recommended that you get this book, especially while it's free!

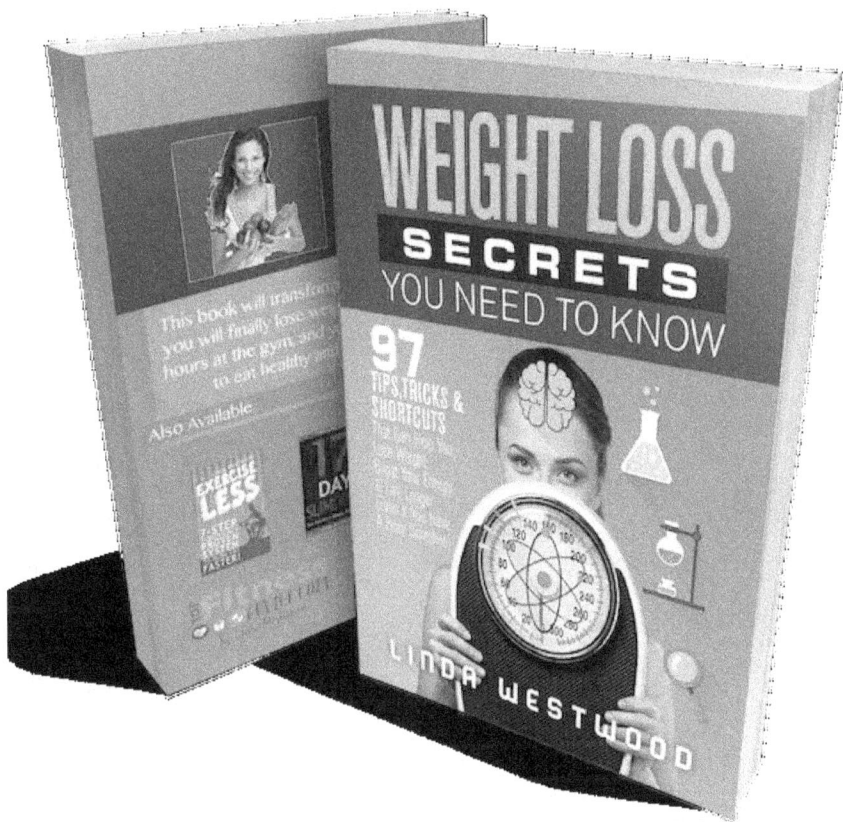

Get Your FREE Copy Here:

TopFitnessAdvice.com/Bonus

Chapter 1

Is It Really Possible?

The title of this book sounds like something of a miracle – 7 Day Total Body Transformation…

This is, after all, what everyone who wants to shift a few extra pounds is longing for – effective weight loss, fast.

But some people would have never come across this amazing dieting concept before, so you may well be asking yourself – is it even possible to "Drop A Dress Size in 7 Days"?

The great news is that, yes, it certainly is!

In this book, we will show you exactly how to carry out this brilliantly effective short-term plan to transform your body in just 7 days. Not just a little, but a considerable change in such a short time – a whole dress size of difference.

This fabulous way to lose weight in just one week is ideal for anyone who wants to look great for an upcoming event.

Perhaps you are planning to go on holiday in a few days and want to maximize your slimming down so that you look spectacular on the beach?

You might be about to have a birthday party or go a company ball or another major social event. You could in fact be a week away from attending a wedding – or even be the bride herself!

Whatever your reasons and motivations, if you want to lose with in just 7 days, this is the diet for you.

You don't have to modify it in weird ways or cross your fingers for luck - if you just follow everything we advise then it WILL definitely work for you, it really is that simple.

What is the Plan?

This 7-day plan is based on eating low-fat, low-calorie, nutrient-rich food.

Starchy carbohydrates are kept to a minimum, but not completely cut out, to encourage better weight loss.

There are 3 meals a day plus two snacks to enjoy, so you really won't go hungry. We will explain exactly how and why this approach works so well in Chapter 3.

Follow the plan just the way we recommend and you will lose enough weight to drop an entire dress size.

What CAN you eat?

You will be amazed at the amount and variety of all the delicious, weight-busting nutrients that can be crammed into only 7 days!

You won't miss out on anything that your body needs and you may even be nourishing yourself much better than normal.

There is a whole lot of fruit, vegetables and fiber, plus healthy lean meat, so you will certainly not be running on empty. In fact, you are likely to enjoy preparing all the simple yet delectable recipes that we have included in this book.

Don't forget, you even get to snack!

Who is this weight loss plan designed for?

This plan is for absolutely anyone who wants to drop a dress size in just 7 days. Or tighten their trouser belt – no reason why guys can't follow the plan too!

If you are looking to shed some weight fast but in a healthy way, then you have chosen the perfect plan.

That said, it is not for everyone without reservation. If you have any underlying health problems or are in any doubt about the suitability of the program for your health situation, please consult your doctor before embarking on this or any weight loss program.

Are there any side effects or downsides?

If you follow the plan exactly, there will be no significant negative effects.

On the contrary, you are likely to be feeling better than ever during and after the 7-day diet!

The only aspect to consider is that this weight loss plan has been especially designed to work quickly and effectively over a short period of time.

It is not meant to be followed in the same way for 6 months, for example.

However, it certainly will be possible to adapt the principles to a longer-term mode of eating once the 7 days are up and we will discuss how later in this book.

Take time to read and absorb that post-plan advice as it will help ensure that you do not gain back any weight.

What do you have to do?

Each day you simply select one breakfast, one lunch and one dinner from the recipes in the later chapters of this book.

You can also enjoy two snacks from the list of ideas outlined in Chapter 9.

In addition, you should not drink anything other than unsweetened herbal tea or water.

We recommend that you aim to drink at least eight glasses of water per day.

Chapter 2

How to Drop a Dress Size!

In this chapter, we take you step by step through the exact way that you can successfully *Drop A Dress Size in 7 Days*. All you have to do is follow these steps.

10 Easy Steps to Help You Drop a Dress Size in 7 Days

1. **Measure Up** - Take a measurement of your body before you begin. Then keep a record of them and see how you measure up after the 7 days.

    BEFORE:

    BUST_____
    _____

    WAIST_____
    _____

    HIPS_____
    _____

    You may already know your dress size, but it is a well-known fact that some clothes shops go bigger or smaller than the official measurement. So, if you want a reliable guide please use the table below as a guide:

US SIZE	BUST		WAIST		HIPS	
	INCHES	CM	INCHES	CM	INCHES	CM
2	31	78.5	23.75	60.5	33.75	86
4	32	81	24.75	63	34.75	88.5
6	34	86	26.75	68	36.75	93.5
8	36	91	28.75	73	38.75	98.5
10	38	96	30.75	78	40.75	103.5
12	40	101	32.75	83	42.75	108.5
14	43	108.5	35.75	90.5	45.75	116

2. **Think about your motivation** – A spot of mental preparation at this stage can make all the difference to your chances of true success.

Think positive, get set, be totally honest and prepare to shine.

Write down your own personal answers to these key questions:

Why am I planning to drop a dress size?

What are the possible pitfalls that I must avoid in order to
maximize the results?

What is my number one aim through doing this program?

Keep a note of your answers to these questions and refer to them during the 7 days if you feel you are starting to lose motivation.

Once you have clarified for yourself why you are going to follow the program, you will find it far easier to motivate yourself.

3. Next, check-off some of the many benefits of losing weight:

- Look totally amazing – slimmer, younger, fitter, healthier and more attractive.

- Dramatically cut your risk of cancer, heart disease, stroke, diabetes and other potentially fatal diseases.

- Get a real buzz from fitting into your favorite smaller-size clothes again, or treating yourself to new ones – it is an outstanding ego boost!

- Start positively vibrating with fresh energy and love being able to enjoy more activities.

- Eliminate toxins from your system with a healthy, low-calorie, low-fat, high-water diet.

- Enjoy glowing skin and a stunning, refreshed complexion.

- Benefit from better digestion – if you have had any internal issues they may simply melt away after the next healthy 7 days.

4. **Browse through the recipes** – Chapters 6 through 10 offer a superb selection of recipes for breakfast, lunch, dinner and snacks and each meal is given its own chapter of recipes.

   Simply pick one breakfast, one lunch, one dinner and two snacks per day.

   There are enough recipes for all 7 days, although if you particularly like one recipe option, please feel free to repeat your choice and eat it another time as well during the week.

   You have to eat them at regular intervals throughout the day, giving yourself at least 3-4 hours between each meal.

5. **Once you have had a chance to review the recipes, take a look at the shopping list and mark off all the ingredients you will need to buy.**

We have not specified strict amounts as that will depend on the choices you make and whether you prefer certain recipes above others.

If you intend to try every single recipe during the 7 days, then simply buy everything on the list – it is all there!

6. Next, go shopping.

Fun!

All you have to do is buy according to the handy list.

However, there is one important additional note to consider when you are shopping. Do aim to buy the best quality fresh ingredients that you can afford.

This does not always have to mean that you buy the most expensive food there is, although we recommend organic options whenever possible and this does tend to come with a higher price tag.

It is always worth buying organic fruit, vegetables, cereals and meat if you can possibly afford it.

It has been widely debated whether eating organic fruit and vegetables is any different to eating regular produce that has been grown with pesticides and other chemicals.

Honestly, it really is different – fact.

Organic fruit and vegetables have been grown in accordance with very strict guidelines to ensure they remain chemical-free. The resulting produce is much higher in antioxidants and much lower in its levels of toxins, metals and pesticides.

Not convinced?

Check out this study by The Organic Trade Association. They found that the significantly higher levels antioxidants in organic crops included:

- 19% higher levels of phenolic acids

- 69% higher levels of flavanones

- 28% higher levels of stilbenes

- 26% higher levels of flavones

- 50% higher levels of flavonols

- 51% higher levels of anthocyanins

All of these antioxidants have been shown to lower the risk of heart disease, brain diseases and certain cancers.

Switch to organic fruit and veg and you will increase the amount of antioxidants you take in by up to 40% - with NO more calories.

That's a great reason to go organic when you grab the Shopping List in Chapter 10!

7. Begin!

Once you have all your, hopefully, organic food, you need to start the plan. Eat the meals according to the guidelines, i.e. 3-4 hours apart and including the two snacks per day.

You can now add a couple more important tips (below and in later chapters) that will turn your week from okay to terrific!

8. Drink a lot of water – Few of us drink as much water as we should to stay healthy, and in fact, many people suffer from dehydration in the majority of their working days.

They drink little water but do not realize why they feel lethargic, or even sick, and find it hard to lose the excess pounds. Water feeds our metabolism and flushes out unhealthy toxins that poison our system.

We need more water in our lives – or specifically in our bodies – to function well. We are made up of 60% water.

We need to keep ourselves constantly topped up with H_2O in order to be able to enjoy the very best of health and lose maximum weight.

So, promise yourself that you will drink at least 8 glasses of water every day during the Drop A Dress Size in 7 Days plan.

Not only will it help you to lose weight, but you will also be blown away by how lovely your skin starts to look.

9. **Keep on movin'** – To maximize the effects of this outstanding weight loss plan, it should be twinned with our special exercise plan.

This plan involves working out at least 4 times during the week, using slowly controlled toning exercises that work your muscles on a deeper level, build strength, and crucially boost your metabolism to the max. We won't outline every exercise that you have to do right here as we go into them in detail in Chapter 4.

Trust us though – you will love them and they will make a real difference.

10. **The 7 Days Are Up!** – Once you have completed the steps for this plan, you will notice a significant difference in how you look and feel compared to the start of the week.

However, the mirror does not always give the full picture; so, make sure you celebrate your transformation by measuring up once more and noting just how much you have lost:

AFTER:

BUST_____

_____

WAIST_____

_____

HIPS_____

_____

Congratulations!

By this point you will have been through everything you need to do to Drop A Dress Size in 7 Days, so all you have to do to enjoy the results to the max...show yourself off, get into those skinny jeans and spread the word about what you have achieved!

I hope that you are enjoying this book so far, and if you could spare 30 seconds, I would greatly appreciate you leaving a review on Amazon.com.

Chapter 3

The SECRET of the Plan

Many people are amazed by this plan. They simply can't believe it is possible. After all, shouldn't losing weight be painful and stressful, with weeks of going hungry and many failed attempts to show for every lost pound?

The answer is a resounding NO!

Once you learn the secret of this plan, it will all become crystal clear.

The plan is not based on chance, luck or superstition.

It is solidly founded on reliable biological principles that will ensure that you get the results that you deserve with this superb diet.

So... What's the Secret?

Okay, since you've asked, let's look at why this diet works every time, when followed corrected.

There are three pillars to this diet.

The low-calorie aspect, the low-fat aspect and the fact that both strategies are supported by calorie-burning, toning exercise.

The trick to understanding why these approaches work is not just to understand each one in isolation, it is to recognize that they get brilliant results when working *in combination.*

In addition to these three pillars, the structure of this diet ensures that your metabolism is kept working at its peak, thanks to thermogenesis and to consuming the right amounts of food that support and promotes a faster metabolism.

How does the structure do this?

Part of the answer lies in the fact that it is essential to eat every 3-4 hours.

In this plan, you never wait too long before the next snack or meal, which has two consequences.

First, you are never tempted to gorge on junk due to hunger.

Second, you are eating at exactly the perfect intervals to keep those metabolic fires burning.

Why Does It Work?

Unless you are an expert in nutrition, it can be hard to understand precisely why the principles of this plan work every time. So, here is some more information outlining why eating this way works so well for weight loss.

The Low-Calorie Factor

If you understand the calorie principle then you will be several steps nearer to controlling your weight for good.

Calories have been discussed in all kinds of ways, but in reality, it is very simple. As time passes throughout a day, we eat a lot of food and at the same time we burn calories every day.

We must also remember that the drinks we drink can also be very high in calories. Alcohol, for example, contains more calories than carbs.

So, taking into account everything that we consume, food and drink alike, whether we gain or lose weight is all simply a question of balance.

If we consume more calories than we burn it will definitely lead to weight gain. If we consume fewer calories than we burn, then we will lose weight.

An average man needs around 2500 calories a day to maintain his weight. For an average woman, that number is around 2000 calories a day.

Some plans recommend that you reduce just 600 calories per day. This is shown to result in anywhere from 1-2lbs of weight loss for a slightly overweight individual.

Obviously, these numbers are all dependent on the individual, what they consume, and how active their lifestyles are.

It is not recommended that anyone consume less than 1000 calories per day when trying to lose weight. But the beauty of this plan is that you do not have to constantly count the calories as we have done that for you.

Losing weight is well worth the effort and not just for looks.

When we carry excess weight, we are at far greater risk of a wide range of serious health problems.

First, when we eat and drink more calories than we need, our bodies store the excess as body fat. Fat can be very dangerous for our health, particularly the extra pounds of fat that so many of us can carry around our belly area.

If this weight gain goes unchecked and continues over time then we will become overweight, and can even become obese.

Being overweight or obese causes an increased risk of type-2 diabetes, heart disease, stroke and some cancers.

Many adults in the US need to lose weight, and to do this they need to eat and drink fewer calories. Combining these changes with increased physical activity is the best way to achieve a healthier weight.

Remember, achieving a healthy weight is all about striking the right balance between the energy that you put into your body, and the energy that you use.

To lose weight, you have to use more energy than you consume in food and drinks throughout the day.

This weight loss book makes this easier for you as it changes your eating habits and encourages physical activity in your daily life. Stick to it strictly for 7 days and you will certainly lose weight.

However, there is much more to it than that. Now let's take a look at the type of calories you will be consuming for 7 days.

Low-fat Food

It makes sense to most people that if you don't want to be fat, then you should probably eat less of it, right?

This is common sense... but it is not the whole story by any stretch of the imagination. There are different types of fats and they act within your body in very different ways...

Everyone needs some fat as the body requires some fat to function properly.

It is a small amount of healthy fat that helps the body to function at optimum levels. But remember the calorie/energy-burning balance.

Fat is very calorie-dense - every gram of fat contains 9 calories. What does that mean? Let's compare it to other macro-nutrients:

Protein: 1 gram = 4 calories

Carbohydrates: 1 gram = 4 calories

Alcohol: 1 gram = 7 calories

Eat too much fat and, at 9 calories per gram, it will obviously be fattening. However, not all fats stack up the same nutritionally and some fats are better for you than others.

Unsaturated Fats

These include both monounsaturated and polyunsaturated fats. Polyunsaturated fats come from plants and include olive oil, corn oil, and canola oil, among others. If you are trying to lose weight you should really stick to this category of fat. You will be pleased to note that the majority of our recipes that require fat specify that you use one of these healthier fats.

Saturated Fats

Saturated fats come from animal products, for example meat and dairy foods. They increase the risk of heart disease because they raise the "bad" LDL cholesterol in the body.

Only 10% or less of your daily calories should be from saturated fats. The American Heart Association recommends even less — 7 percent.

However, this is as part of a normal, daily maintenance diet. If you are trying to actually lose weight then of course it should be far less if possible.

Trans Fats

Quite simply, these are the worst types of fats to eat and too many of them can impact hugely on our health.

Trans fats can be found in products like margarines as well as in many unhealthy snacks such as processed foods including cookies, cakes, pies, ready meals and potato chips.

Trans fats come in many disguises but they are basically created when liquid oils are transformed into more solid fats, sometimes called "partially hydrogenated oils".

This is commonly done to increase the shelf life of packaged food and it is a dangerous feature of processed, packaged, unhealthy foods.

Trans fats can actually raise your bad cholesterol and as such, many medical experts recommend that you avoid them altogether.

Why A Low-Fat Diet Works?

On a low-fat diet, you restrict your calorie intake through fat to a lower than normal percentage. For example, on a normal weight-loss diet of 1,200 calories, you will limit fats to only 20% of total daily intake.

This basically means that you can have 240 calories, or 26 grams, of fat each day, with a maximum of 120 calories, or 13 grams, coming from saturated fat. That leaves you with nearly a full 1,000 calories to "consume" on protein and carbohydrates.

However, this plan is no ordinary diet.

For a start, we encourage the consumption of some low-fat dairy products. They are rich in calcium and vitamin D and these helps preserve and build muscle mass.

The higher the percentage of fat in your body and the less muscle, the worse your ability to burn calories. Conversely, having a good muscle mass is essential for maintaining a super-efficient metabolism.

We also recommend that, in order for this superb weight-loss program to work at its best in a short space of time – you eat less than the standard amount of even the healthy fats.

This way you will be burning stores of unwanted fat to make up the difference, which you will be hugely grateful for when you see how great you look after just a few days!

Not to Forget... The Thermogenic Factor!

Certain foods have a very high thermogenic effect, so you literally torch away the calories as you eat. Other foods contain nutrients and compounds that add kindling to your metabolic fire. Feed your metabolism with these wonderful dietary additions.

- **Whole grains:** When your body tries to break down whole foods your body burns twice as many calories.

  This is especially true when it comes to those foods that are rich in fiber, like oatmeal and brown rice.

If you only consume processed foods, you lose this advantage, as well as lots of fiber and vital nutrients.

- **Lean meats:** Lean protein really is the dieters' friend and it has a very high thermogenic effect.

Did you know that you burn about 30% of the calories the food contains during digestion?

This means that a 300-calorie chicken breast requires about 90 calories to break it down. Eat lean and burn, baby, burn!

- **Lentils:** One cup of lentils packs in an amazing 35% of your daily iron needs. This is fabulous news, since up to 20% of us are iron- deficient.

When you lack a nutrient, your metabolism slows down because the body's not getting everything that it needs to work efficiently and to lose weight, your body needs to be working as efficiently as possible.

- **Hot peppers:** Want to add some real fire to your metabolism and burn calories as efficiently as possible? Capsaicin, the compound that gives chili peppers their heat, warms up your body, so that you burn off additional calories. You can get it by eating raw, cooked, dried, or powdered peppers.

Some of our brilliant recipes include a little chili, or if not, you can up your burn rate simply by nibbling a tiny raw chili pepper alongside your chosen food.

- **Green tea:** It is a proven fact that green tea can help you dramatically lose weight, more than any other drink (apart from water).

  Drinking four cups of green tea a day, helped people shed more than six pounds in eight weeks, as it was reported following a study in the American Journal of Clinical Nutrition.

  There is a compound in the green tea called EGCG and it temporarily speeds metabolism after sipping it. To up your intake, keep a jug of iced tea in the fridge.

- **Fabulous Fish:** Salmon is high in protein, and a fatty fish such as salmon contains essential omega-3 fatty acids. These have been shown to regulate a vital body hormone called leptin, which is involved in the regulation of energy.

  When leptin is efficiently regulated and present in the body in lower levels, this hormone an associated with an increased caloric burn. Tuna is also an excellent source of omega-3s and should freely be enjoyed as part of a healthy diet.

The Carbs Question

On the weight loss plan, we include reduced levels of wheat intake. This means less white bread and pasta - for several reasons.

First, starchy carbohydrate acts just like sugar in the body, spiking the blood and causing a surge of insulin... The result? The body is commanded to hold onto the calories as fat. Not good!

In this diet, the starchy carbs, things including but not limited to bread, noodles and pasta, potatoes, root vegetables like parsnips, and rice, are strictly limited.

This is with good reason as they are not only calorie-dense, but they will simply cause you to feel bloated and are converted straight into fat if you eat too them in great quantities (and aren't able to burn the resulting energy).

On the flip side, if you cut them out completely, then you can find that you simply put weight straight back on when you start eating them again.

We want your weight loss to be both highly effective and lasting, so we encourage you to enjoy light amounts of carbs as part of this diet. You will find that this helps to curb your hunger and also keeps your metabolism burning.

Staying Off the Caffeine

Throughout the 7-day period, you also need to avoid all alcohol and caffeine.

Alcohol is bad for dieting all round, as it is very high in calories at 7 calories per gram, plus is drains your energy, acts as a depressant and hampers your metabolism.

Additionally, you will be exercising regularly and this is terrible for your health if you try to do it under the influence of alcohol (or have any traces of alcohol in your blood)!

Also, during the 7-day diet do not drink regular coffee or tea at all as these are packed with caffeine, which we all know is a stimulant. Despite being great in some instances, for the goal we have for these 7 days it won't be that great of a help.

However, herbal infusions and rooibos/red bush tea are absolutely fine. Naturally, you should also make sure that you avoid all energy drinks as they are simply packed with added sugar, often labeled under other names like 'glucose' and so on.

You Will NOT Starve

By this stage you should have taken a look at all the recipes in this book. We hope the variety and great tastes on offer have come as a pleasant surprise!

After all, the meals in this plan are not designed to starve you skinny. The length of this diet may be short, but the results are meant to be more than short-term.

Starving will only backfire because you will be hungry and miserable all the time and more likely to eat unhealthy snacks or overdo the portion sizes. You should note that when you starve-eat-starve-eat your body goes into total crisis mode and it immediately stores fat. It is a survival response – we were not meant to starve.

Our poor bodies do not know we are aiming to look thinner and does its best to hold onto every single calorie, so the cruel result is that you pack on a load of extra weight, so you starve again and the cycle goes on and on...

This slimming plan is completely different. It is low in fat and low in calories, so the weight comes of quickly, very quickly, but it does not starve you to an unhealthy degree, so your body thrives rather that fights to survive.

You will not starve on this diet. Remember, you will be eating two snacks a day in addition to three full meals per day and your body really does not need more than that if you follow our recipes.

On the contrary, this weight loss plan will not give you too much or too little of anything – you will receive just enough to *drop a dress size in 7 days*, period.

Consuming all those empty calories in sugary, fatty or processed foods will not trip you up.

However, you will certainly not starve either - you will receive all the best nutrients and plenty of fiber and water. Your digestion will function properly, you will burn plenty of calories and your metabolic rate, boosted by the exercise you are doing, will even increase.

Stick to the program for 7 days and the pounds will fall off.

The Water Secret

You are advised to drink a lot of water throughout the 7-day slimming program.

And it will work wonders for your weight loss, skin, digestion and general health.

If you drink little and often, you will find it easier.

Try starting your day with a refreshing, rehydrating, detoxifying, cleansing, enjoyable glass of water and lemon.

Keep a bottle of water with you wherever you go.

Drink some peppermint tea after your evening meal (it is wonderful for digestion) and try to end the day with more water, perhaps in the form of another soothing herbal tea like chamomile. Water has an amazing amount of benefits for the body.

First, it keeps you completely hydrated, which is absolutely vital for your body to function properly. Water also flushes out the vast majority of toxins and it does it healthily and effectively.

Plus, it keeps your metabolism all fired up and your digestion working at its peak, two benefits that are the best possible news for anyone who is trying to lose weight.

There is even more good news when it comes to drinking plenty of water. Water fills you up brilliantly so that you are far less tempted to cheat with fatty or calorific snacks.

It also fully quenches your thirst, whereas alcohol, coffee and sodas, even diet sodas, just pretend to, while dehydrating you even more - and best of all water contains zero calories.

Have a love affair with water throughout the whole of the next 7 days and afterwards as well. Try to drink 6-8 large glasses each day.

Chapter 4

Speed Up Your Transformation

Now that you are getting closer to beginning your transformation of a whole dress size – it is time to consider that other pillar of weight loss success. That's right, the exercise factor.

Almost anyone who has lost weight, however much and however quickly, has explained that it has, in some respect, been down to eating less and moving more.

This slimming plan is no different in that regard. In fact, it focuses on exercise even more carefully than usual as you only have a week to play with.

So, what is the most effective form of exercise to change your body shape and burn ample calories in just 7 days?

Is it doing 20 crunches, going for a walk, or jogging?

No, no and no – they are all great forms of exercise, but for this program we need exercises that will create a long, deep calorie-burn and work your muscles effectively.

Plus, the whole workout has to be more compact because life is busy and there may not be time to excrcise for one or two hours every day.

A current workout that has proven very popular and effective relies on carrying out different exercises intensively but for just 90 seconds.

That's right, just a minute and a half of work, but each exercise is so well-targeted that it can make a whole of difference to your body

How Does the 90-Second Workout Work?

The fun thing about the 90-Second Workout is that instead of doing 30 press-ups or 40 crunches over and over, you do each exercise just once, or once on each side. Unbelievable!

To make it work, you spread the movements over 90 seconds, even though it is just one rep, so that the muscles work really hard to tighten and tone your physique.

So – one long rep instead of 20 or 30. Sounds totally doable, right? Well it is – and it is also fun and very effective indeed.

Follow this routine for the first 3 days of the plan. Then, have Day 4 off, then do the routine again on Day 5, Day 6 and Day 7.

Safety First

A few notes before you start exercising. While this routine is designed to help you, it is important not to stress your body to the extent that you do yourself an injury.

If you are not currently fit, or if you currently have an injury of any kind, please consult your doctor. If in doubt it would be better to delay following the plan until you are given permission to continue by a medical professional.

The Exercises

There are just four main postures to carry out in this routine, although some exercises are comprised of a couple of parts. They will work your body deeply, burn calories and build muscular strength... which means you will burn even more calories.

Muscle tissue burns more calories than fat, even when you are resting. According to scientists, 10 pounds of fat burns 20 calories when you are resting, while 10 pounds of muscle in a person of the same size burns 50 calories.

Exercise is quite simply the gift that keeps on giving!

Exercise 1 – The Super-Squat

This exercise works the legs and butt to perfection.

To achieve the initial position, stand with your feet shoulder-width apart and your arms raised to shoulder height, balancing carefully.

Slowly bend your knees and lower your body, being careful to keep your hips over your heels and your back straight.

When you have reached one-third of the way down, pause and hold your position for a full 10 seconds.

Carry on descending 2 inches, lower 2 inches, raising your heels if you need to. Hold this position for a further 10 seconds. Repeat this lowering and holding technique three more times, each time keeping position for a full 10 seconds.

Note: Make sure you hold your belly in and keep your shoulders back as you perform this exercise. It will make a lot of difference.

Exercise 2 – Backwards Fly with Ball

This exercise may seem difficult at first but don't give up. It is really worth mastering this move as it thoroughly works the thighs, butt, back, arms and shoulders. There are two parts to this exercise. You will need two dumbbells weighing 5 to 8 pounds and a medium to large sized exercise ball.

1. Begin with one dumbbell in each hand and your right leg lifted behind you so that the top of your right foot rests on the exercise ball behind you.

    Bend your left knee to 45 degrees, rolling the exercise ball backward and hinging forward until your back is parallel to the floor and your arms are hanging straight down.

2. With your elbows slightly bent, raise each arm a few inches and hold the position for 10 seconds.

Then raise your arms 2 inches more, and hold for another 10 seconds. Repeat this pattern of lifting and holding 3 more times, until you end with your arms at shoulder height.

Then slowly lower your arms a few inches, hold for 10-seconds and do this 3 more times.

Now repeat the whole exercise standing on the other leg.

Note: It will help you a great deal if you draw your abs in and up and keep your hips square. Don't worry if you wobble, just regain your balance and keep going.

Exercise 3 - Ab-Fab Rotations

This exercise is performed lying down, but don't be fooled into think this is some kind of rest!

1. Lie down on your back with your legs lifted straight up. Your arms should reach out to either side with your palms down.

2. Lower both your legs a few inches to the left, then hold that pose for a full 10 seconds. Lower your left 2 inches more to the left, and then hold for another 10 seconds.

   Repeat the lowering and holding 3 more times, until you end up you're your legs hovering just above the floor. Raise your legs back to the center in 4 increments, raising and then holding for 10 seconds each time.

Now repeat the whole exercise on the opposite side.

Note: Make sure you keep your abs drawn in as you move, to protect your lower back and also keep your right shoulder down to prevent strain.

If you want to mix things up a bit, you can also try rotating your legs left and holding them just a few inches from the floor for a full 45 seconds. Then return to the top position and repeat the hold on the right side.

Exercise 4 - Fly the Bridge Backwards

This outstanding exercise is not always easy at first but persevere as it is worth getting right. It works the hips, hamstrings, butt, chest, arms, and shoulders, so it is a pretty comprehensive exercise all-round. You will need the dumbbells and the exercise ball once again.

1. Lie flat on your back with your feet on top of the exercise ball and your legs straight, being careful not to lock your knees.

   Hold a dumbbell in each hand, with your arms raised over your chest. Press your heels into the ball, and slowly lift your hips so that your body forms a straight line.

   Do try and keep it as straight as possible as your hips may be tempted to sag – don't let them!

2. Bend your elbows slightly, then open your arms a few inches to the side; hold this position for a full 10 seconds.

   Open your arms 2 inches more, and hold again for10 seconds. Repeat this opening and holding 3 more times. Then close your arms in 4 increments, each time with holding period that lasts 10 seconds.

Note: This is not the easiest, but it is worth it. Don't worry if you need to take a quick break partway through. Just stop, breathe deeply and get going again as soon as you are able.

Time Out

That's it, you're done. This set of exercises will really reach the parts that other workouts can't reach, so expect to feel like you have worked hard.

However, it has only taken a few minutes to achieve some serious muscle flexing and calorie burning. Now just unwind and look forward to repeat the routine every day, apart from Day 4 of the plan.

Don't forget to share your thoughts on this book by leaving a review on Amazon.com.

Chapter 5

Top Tips to Drop a Dress Size FAST

So – you know what food you are about to start eating and why.

You know the right exercises to perform and how.

You have a water bottle on standby.

You are feeling positive, motivated and excited.

But here's the thing – there are only 7 days to drop the weight, so what other things can you do to turbo-charge your weight loss and achieve maximum results?

Read on, you might be surprised...

1. Try to minimize your sugar and carb intake as much as possible.

They may be the first 'treats' we all reach for when we are stressed, upset or tired and as they tend to be highly processed and packaged we don't usually even have to go to the trouble of cooking them ourselves.

Sugary snacks and too many carbs really are your enemies for the duration of this diet. You may feel you need them, but you don't – they may give you a sugar rush, but you will feel horrible when you crash back down to earth.

If only for 7 days, just don't do it, it's not worth it. That is not to say you can never ever eat a donut again, of course you can. But after dropping a dress size and looking better than ever you may not even want to anytime soon.

2. Make sweat your friend

That's right, time to really sweat. We have looked at the exercises and if you do those right then you should certainly get pretty worked out, but you can sweat even more than that!

Time to rediscover the pleasures of a great session in a sauna, or even to try it for the first time. You may already know that our skin is our largest organ and largely responsible, along with our liver and kidneys, for the elimination of toxins.

We need to appreciate our ability to sweat and make the most of it. After all, sweat contains measurable amounts of toxins that have been safely removed from the tissues.

When you sweat, you are detoxifying your body and when you do that, it encourages weight loss.

We know that sweating is good for us. When it doesn't occur in a situation that we find socially embarrassing, we can even relax and feel the impurities being drawn out of us, a wonderful feeling of being cleansed.

Sweating helps clear out nasty toxins and excess fluid and can be a great starting point for a healthier lymphatic system and a faster metabolism.

So, why don't we spending more time sweating our troubles away?

Well, not everyone has a sauna at home, or even in their nearest gym. But during this 7-day program, it would be great if you could have at least two sauna sessions.

Some people also find the high temperatures uncomfortable. However, they should be aware that there are now many more low temperature saunas.

A typical sauna is anywhere from 160 – 180°F, but the less common "thermal chambers" are set to around 100 – 120°F, so you can realistically stay in there for much longer than the usual 15 minutes or so and therefore you will sweat more.

More sweat means more depuration, or washing away of toxins. The toxins essentially get carried away by the water that our body produces, like rivers washing dirt and litter away. Sweat works in the same way.

So, do enjoy the pleasures of a good sauna. If you can, try to line one up after you do your exercise routine, as you will sweat even more. Alternatively, go straight from the office and relax in the heat – the important thing is just to sweat!

Saunas can play a really important part of any diet or detox regime. They will only boost your progress and make you feel good. Just make sure you remember to shower thoroughly afterwards, before you simply reabsorb the unwanted toxins.

3. Detox to the max

A key reason why your body is holding excess fluid and extra fat is due to a build-up of harmful toxins.

Modern life is pretty toxic, so it can be pretty hard to avoid coming into contact with substances that poison our system – skin creams, cosmetics, alcohol, medicines and drugs, detergents, perfumes... we are bombarded with toxins every day, even before we take a mouthful of food that contains, pesticides, additives, preservatives and other dubious, potentially carcinogenic substances.

If you smoke as well, it is at least ten times as damaging...

Wouldn't it be great to stem the endless flow of toxins, even for just one week?

Well you can, as much as possible – view this 7-day plan as an opportunity.

Drink the recommended amounts of water (starting the day with water and lemon), do the exercises and follow the diet closely as discussed – this will all help detoxify your system.

But on top of that you can add in not only saunas but also something called dry skin brushing to physically move the toxins out of your system.

4. Dry body brushing

The benefits of dry skin brushing include increasing the circulation to the skin and therefore reducing the appearance of cellulite.

Skin looks smoother, brighter and clearer. Dry skin brushing may also help rid the body of annoying ingrown hairs.

However, the main point of this activity is to detoxify the body.

Dry skin brushing helps to hugely improve blood circulation and lymphatic drainage. It releases toxins and promotes the discharge of metabolic waste.

Also, dry skin can clog the pores and therefore brushing dead skin cells away helps your skin to absorb nutrients in a far more efficient manner.

All this means that after a little dry brushing the body can function more effectively. In turn, this means that you can lose weight much more quickly!

Enjoy a better detoxification and simply get into a routine of dry brushing every morning before your shower or bath. It is very straightforward, does not take much time and you don't need membership of some exclusive spa.

All you need to do is buy a natural bristle brush with a long handle so you will be able to reach all areas of the body.

Here's exactly how you do it:

- Take your brush and work it around your body in gentle circular, upward motions, followed by longer, smoother strokes.

- When you perform a dry body brush, always start at your ankles and work upwards in slow firm movements towards the heart. There is a logical reason for this - the lymphatic fluid (which critically fights infection and disease) flows through the body towards the heart. It is therefore very important that you move the brush in the same direction.

- There is one exception to this rule which applies to your back. Brush in firm strokes from the neck down to the lower back.

- From your ankles, slowly move up to your calves and then brush your knee area, thighs, stomach, back and arms. Do not brush too hard over the softer and more sensitive areas of skin located around the chest and breasts. Also, make sure that you never brush over inflamed or broken skin, sunburn, or skin cancer.

- When you have given your body a thoroughly good brushing always jump straight into the nearest shower in order to wash away all those dead skin cells and harmful released toxins. Remember, leave toxins on your skin for too long and they will simply be reabsorbed into your system.

- Top tip: If you would like to stimulate the skin even more and invigorate your blood circulation, then play around with the temperature of the shower. Turn the control from hot to cold and cold to hot a few times, which will not only give your pores a work out that tingles, it will also make you feel really alive!

- After you have showered, do apply a wonderful, rich and nourishing moisturizer to your damp skin. Do keep it unfragranced and as natural as possible if you can, otherwise what was the point of all that detoxing? For best results use pure cocoa butter, or coconut oil, while argan oil is outstanding for problem areas like scars or stretch marks.

- Repeat the dry brushing routine as often as you like. If you keep it up for each of the 7 days and then carry on afterwards you will transform the quality of your skin as well as your body,]

5. De-stress

Question: Is the rumor that stress makes you fat actually true?

Answer: It certainly is!

Why exactly does stress make you fat?

It is something that feels as if it is true and we have all had those days when we have been over-burdened or strung out and eaten exactly the wrong thing because it was hot, quick and greasy.

That is one way that stress makes us fat – we are unhappy and so we eat to soothe our emotions rather than to fuel us with nutrients. Or more accurately we overeat to soothe our emotions...

Plus, when we grab that burger, it is not just high-calorie and high-fat, it is also high in sodium. Sodium, or salt, causes you to retain water and it is found in large quantities in highly processed or fast foods.

However, there is even more to it than that. Stress itself can also cause you to hold onto fluid, making you feel constantly puffy and bloated, not a great feeling at all.

Finally, stress leads to the production of hormones that slower your metabolism and reduce the speed of weight loss.

So how can you get rid of stress?

In several ways:

- *Consider meditation.* This ancient form of deep relaxation can be very therapeutic and is highly recommended for people who are feeling stressed or who suffer from what can be described as 'a chatty mind'.

- *Write a journal at the end of every day.* Unburdening your main of the day's events can feel very rewarding and reassuring.

Do it long-hand with a pen rather than online in order to relax properly as the light emitted from computer screens and other devices can cause insomnia.

Conversely, writing in the old-fashioned way is relaxing and sharing your troubles, secrets and thoughts with a confidential book is very soothing indeed.

- *Face the problem.* If you have a specific issue that is making you stressed, face it head-on before attempting a weight loss program.

Share your troubles with a partner, co-worker or friend, or even simply write a list of the issues with ideas about how to tackle it. It the problem is a real biggie that can't be addressed in a week, you can still take positive steps.

Contact someone who can help – a doctor, lawyer or therapist. Get an appointment in the diary and a load will be lifted from your shoulders.

6. Ditch the salt habit

We have touched upon this when looking at stress – too much sodium in the diet can lead directly to water retention, which means a puffy, bloated body.

Not good.

What is good is the fact that you hold the solution in your hands, literally.

Put down the salt for a week. It will not add calories, but it will add to the amount of water that you ultimately retain, so who needs it?

You can still season your food and you will be surprised how much flavors can be enhanced by other herbs like parsley and coriander, or spices like cumin, or the brightest flavor hit of all - a little squeeze of lime and a couple of thin slices of chili – delicious!

7. Care for the inner you

No one ever succeeded in a weight loss plan without a clear idea in their own mind about why they are doing it in the first place. We have touched upon this in the earlier preparation stages but it really is worth re-emphasizing.

Get your head straight.

Dig deep, give yourself a little tough love... whatever it takes. Keep a note on you at all times that reads:

"I am doing this because _____"

It could be something simple like "because I have a wedding to go to next Saturday" or it could be something much deeper. It doesn't matter, it's not a writing competition. It's all about you, so make it honest and make it personal to you.

Pay attention to your state of mind during the 7 days. If you feel you are getting down, take steps to pep yourself up, with a beauty treat, going to see a movie, or just having a good chat with a friend.

If you are in great shape in your head you can get into great shape in terms of your body.

8. Favor only the good fats

Healthy omega-3 fats can help you lose weight.

Linseed, walnuts, mackerel and sardines among other foods all help produce the fat-burning enzyme PPAR-alpha. This enzyme is known to help prevent the storage of fat on the body.

Be very sure to understand this – eating a little good, natural fat will not result in piling on the pounds. However, in this low-calorie, low-fat diet, even the good fats are to be consumed in moderation.

9. Start the plan on a Thursday

Sounds strange perhaps, but research proves that you're twice as likely to stick to a diet when you get nearer to the weekend.

The pressure is off but the motivation is on, so boost your willpower and forget the tyranny of Manic Mondays for good!

10. Laugh it up!

Just when you thought we were getting too serious...

This is a little reminder that getting slim and gorgeous really is fun!

The diet plan is fantastic and that, along with the exercise, will help you drop a dress size, but you can make certain lifestyle changes that may help.

Laughing properly, with deep 'belly laughs' - are exactly that; they work and strengthen your abdominal muscles.

Think about it – that has to be the most fun workout ever!

Still, life isn't always a barrel of laughs, so you can't be expected to be constantly rolling around in a state of mirth. But you can stay upbeat, be more open to laughter and encourage the release of those stress-busting endorphins that come with a good chuckle.

There seems to be a pattern forming here when it comes to getting the right state of mind for weight loss and it appears to be 'don't worry, be happy'!

11. Focus on your food

Don't be confused – this does not mean worrying about more creative food ideas – we have all that covered for you in later chapters.

But it does mean that you should concentrate on what you're eating, when you are eating it.

Don't eat in front of the TV, don't eat on the run and definitely don't shovel food into your mouth at the cinema without thinking... It's time to be mindful about what you eat.

Sit and eat at the table, the old-fashioned way. It has lots of advantages, not least making you realize in both body and mind that you are eating. Dress up the table if you like. Put away your smartphone. Chew properly and take your time.

It will be worth it – studies who that people who eat while texting or watching TV may overindulge by up to 30%. Chances are they are so engrossed in the movie that they don't even realize what they are doing!

So – focus on your food. You will eat far less and enjoy it much, much more.

12. Get green power

There are certain health supplements that you can take which may help you lose weight. Seek these ultra-healthy supplements out at your nearest health-food shop to boost you 7-day plan.

They tend to work by either speeding up your metabolism or cleansing your body of even more toxins:

Green coffee – This contains a caffeinc-based ingredient that speeds up fat metabolism so you lose weight quicker.

Spirulina – This is a type of micro-algae that can be used to maximize the detox effects of the Drop a Dress Size in 7 Days plan. It is a super-effective and healing detoxifying agent which taste like harmless vegetable matter and comes in powder form.

Chlorella - Natural superfood chlorella has exceptional detoxifying properties that help to eliminate mercury and other toxins. It also comes in powdered form, you can mix it with the spirulina powder and add water, the drink it down for a pre-breakfast detox boost.

Green tea – Don't forget to keep drinking this to give a boost to your metabolism.

Flax seeds – Not technically green, but still plant-based so they count. Flaxseeds contain many highly beneficial nutrients, including vitamins, minerals, omega-3 fatty acids and fiber, which normalize the work of the intestine.

Flax absorbs the toxic compounds from the food, cleans the intestines and supplies the body with lecithin, which stimulates the metabolism of fat.

Not bad for a few little seeds!

Sprinkle them raw over some of the delicious dishes in the recipe section for added crunch, taste and most importantly a whole lot more nutritional and detox power.

13. Don't hate your scales.

You may be measuring in inches and your dress size, but if you are determined to lose weight, you will need to start thinking of your scale as a friend, not an enemy.

Weigh yourself once a day, first thing in the morning after going to the bathroom and getting undressed. This way your numbers will not be swayed by water weight and clothing – every pound counts.

A week is a short time, but if you track your results and stay motivated you may be amazed how the pounds can come off quickly.

14. Embrace the power of positive thinking.

Post little notes with your goals written on them in spots you'll see, especially on the fridge.

Other good places include the top of your computer screen and the bathroom mirror – wherever you will spend some time looking each day.

Write what you want to do and why, for example:

"I want to drop a dress size in 7 days so I look great at my best friend's wedding."

Make it short, clear and honest. Research conducted by the Dominican University of California showed that people who wrote down their goals, shared them with a friend, and then followed up with weekly updates were, on average, 33% more successful than those who didn't write down their goals or share them with others.

You may only have a week but stay motivated every day and beyond by writing down your goals.

15. Don't be tempted to skip

If you are going to succeed on this 7-day plan, you have to trust it. Stick to it just as it is written and you will lose weight.

You may think that it would be quicker and more effective to take a shortcut, in other words, by skipping the odd breakfast or lunch.

Our advice?

Don't do it.

You may end up taking in fewer calories that say, but you will also have slowed your metabolism back down and, if you go for too many hours without eating, you may even have kicked your body into starvation mode.

You really do not want to do that, as it is in this mode that the body hold onto every single calorie for dear life and stores as much fat as possible, just in case the body won't receive any food for a while.

So – don't skip breakfast, lunch, or dinner and eat both your snacks. Your appetite will be sated, you won't cheat on the diet and your metabolism will not slow down, jeopardizing your diet.

16. Get app happy

You don't need to do this to succeed in this diet plan, but if you are a lover of tech and are glued to your smartphone anyway, you may find it motivating and fun...

Track your calories with a great app such as My Fitness Pal. You can even scan barcodes that will tell you the precise amount of calories, although as you are eating fresh that will hopefully be on a packet of carrots rather than a bag of pretzels.

Calorie-counting may lose its novelty after 7 days, but if you love your stats and want to see reports that show how much energy more energy you are burning than consuming, try an app like this one.

17. Ban the booze, period

This is one that many dieters dread, but it is very important. Do not be tempted to have a glass of wine, or a beer, under any circumstances during the 7-day plan. Alcohol is simply too calorific, plus it is a toxin and it will stop you from exercising properly.

In addition to that it may weaken your willpower and encourage cravings for high-salt, high-fat foods...Bad news for dieters all round.

Give your liver a break and just ditch the booze, totally and willingly, for the whole week.

Some people who worry about this tip more than any other report back afterwards and have no idea what they were worried about.

You really can go liquor-free for a few days. Then, when you are feeling fresh and great, you will simply wonder why you didn't do it sooner!

18. Look for ways to fidget.

Researchers discovered that people who tap their feet, fidget, and move around more burn 350 extra calories a day—that's more than a major fast-food joint's cheeseburger!

If you do not fidget naturally, just keep one getting up and moving around throughout the day, stretch, jump, bounce and dance around your home, to increase your calorie burn rate throughout the day.

19. Move around the office more.

You may be stuck at a desk for the vast majority of the day, but you can still make calorie-burning differences with a few small changes to your behavior:

Ditch emails on Friday: Change the habits of a working lifetime and walk over to your colleagues instead as once used to happen in every office, when everyone was slimmer!

If you are in a big office this is all the more reason to do it, you might really clock up some miles.

Use a standing desk: A modern solution to the problem that millions of us who are stuck at a desk all day face. Essentially, this higher-level desk is designed to be used while standing, which keeps you more active, toned and burning more calories as well.

Alternatively...

Sit down but use a Desk Stepper: This is a clever machine that is becoming increasing popular and is quite widely available. It simply goes under your desk while you remain seated.

It works like a stair stepper and you tread on it while you do your normal day's work. The beauty of this is that it is not as conspicuous as a standing desk, but will still work off a decent number of calories – over 90 in 20 minutes.

Well worth investing in this little piece of kit when you add up how much you could lose over a week.

Have active meetings: If your schedule includes lots of sitting through meetings every day, change it up. If just two of you are having an internal chat, well why not agree that you will stroll as you talk.

You can cover some ground and it might even keep you more switched on and inspired for longer as the blood gets moving around.

Make it a fitness-friendly office: Don't sit among a bank of computer screen with everything at arms' length like most of us do. Try shaking things up a bit so that you simply have to move to carry out your job.

Of course, you may be busy, but fit, active people get more done in the long run, so it is worth the extra effort. One small example would be to move your trash right away from you so you have to walk back and forth to your desk.

Better still, get rid of it altogether so that you have to go to another part of the building entirely. You may be astounded at how much office carpet you cover with this move. It does pay dividends.

Have many water cooler moments: Don't sit with a huge bottle of mineral water at your desk. No, we are not suggesting that you keeping topping up with gallons of coffee instead!

Keep a small glass handy and keep getting up to refill it at the water cooler which is hopefully a bit of a walk away. This might sound like a waste of time, but it is in fact a clever way of building in the regular breaks from your desks that doctors and health professionals agree are much better for your continued health.

Plus, it has other benefits too – you will keep yourself hydrated with nice, cool, fresh water and you are highly unlikely to miss out on any of the best office gossip for which the water cooler has deservedly become so famous!

Get a Park Buddy: At lunchtime, don't be tempted to hide behind your screen eating a sandwich and sitting still for the fourth hour in a row. Why not ask a friend if they would like to get some fresh air with you in the local park?

It might just be that you go for a casual stroll or a brisk walk, or you might play some sports there even simply jumping after a Frisbee (great exercise) – whatever makes you happy and gets you moving.

Enjoying this book?

Check out my other best sellers!

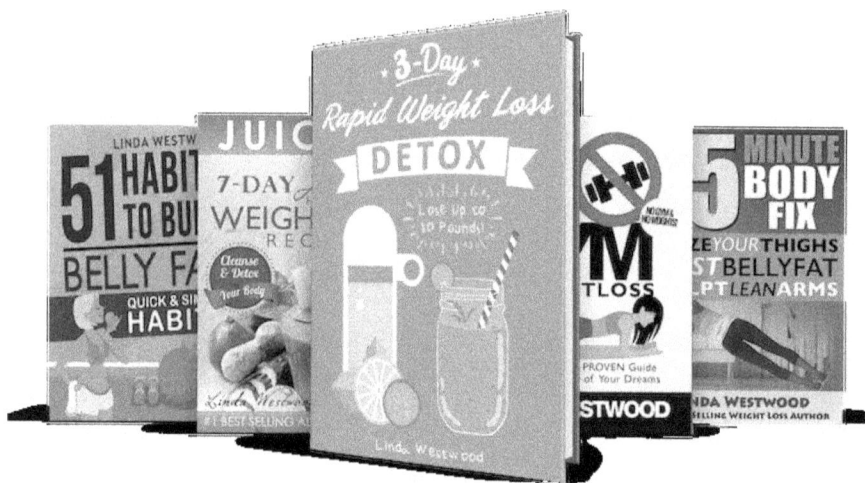

Get your next book on sale here:

TopFitnessAdvice.com/go/books

Chapter 6

Breakfast Recipes

The phrase 'A Breakfast of Champions' is worth remembering as the fittest and most active people tend to swear by eating a good morning meal to set them up for the day.

Breakfast revs up our internal engines and fires up our metabolism so that we burn calories more quickly for the rest of the day – provided we eat the right food.

It is vital to choose the best options first thing in the morning. After all we are literally breaking our fast after a night of sleep and our bodies are crying out for the right fuel and hydration.

The first thing you should consume upon waking is a large glass of still, warm or room temperature water with a slice of lemon in it.

That will hydrate and refresh you beautifully, as well as helping to cleanse and detoxify your system.

Next comes breakfast. But what do you eat when you want to Drop A Dress Size in 7 Days?

We have made it super-simple for you. Just pick one of the 7 breakfast recipes in this chapter and prepare it just as we instruct. Then you will receive the perfectly balance of calories and nutrients in low-fat form.

The recipes are so quick, easy and delicious, you will probably keep on making these breakfasts after the 7 days are up!

We have consciously only given you the 7 best recipes that we could devise, so that life remains far simpler and you don't have to browse through page after page, building a super-long shopping list.

Just choose one recipe per day and if you come across one that you are not keen on, just repeat one of the other recipes. The official Shopping List in Chapter 10 states all the ingredients that you will need.

Whatever you do, don't ever be tempted to skip your nutritious breakfast. A number of respected studies prove the link between obesity and people skipping breakfast.

Conversely, people who are trying to lose weight are more likely to succeed when they eat a good, healthy breakfast. You can't get healthier than these low-calorie, low-fat meals, which also punch well above their weight in terms of taste.

Enjoying a good breakfast will not only fuel your metabolism, it will give you the energy to exercise properly.

The workout you will be performing on most days will be most effective when you are well hydrated and nourished – and breakfast eaters exercise more effectively.

Also, when you eat a decent breakfast you are less likely to 'cheat' on your diet as you won't feel hungry.

While starving ourselves can sometimes seem like a short cut, it rarely is because the body responds in the end by clinging on to its fat stores, making it much harder to lose the unwanted weight...

There is never any need to skip a meal during the diet, so simply relax, browse the recipes and enjoy your great breakfast. It will ultimately help you to look and feel fantastic!

Very Berry Muesli

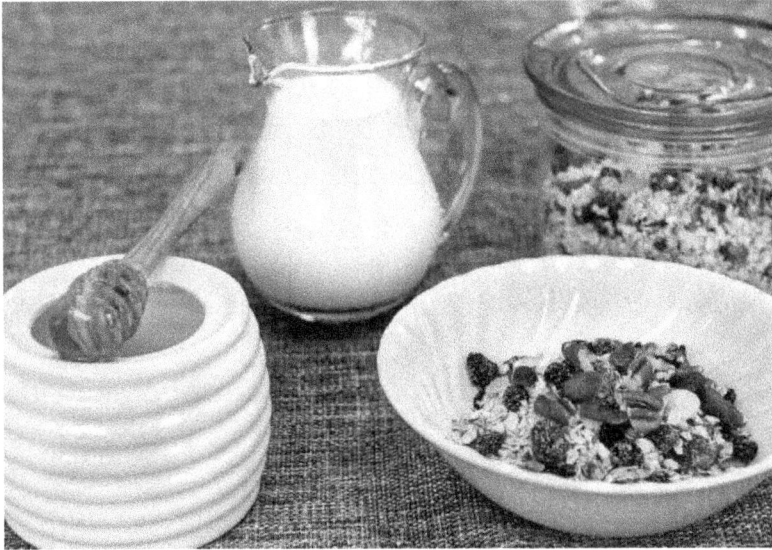

Muesli can make a great breakfast, particularly when it is the coarse, unsweetened kind, which goes heavy on the wholegrain and heart-healthy oats.

It provides slow-burning fuel and will keep you feeling satisfied until lunchtime for relatively few calories.

Meanwhile, the fat-free natural yoghurt delivers outstanding health benefits. The calcium boost will support excellent bone health, which is great news at any age.

Also, a respected study showed that dieters who ate some yogurt daily lost more belly fat, and retained more lean muscle than those in the same study who did not eat yogurt, so eat up.

Finally, the raspberries are a superb fruit addition, providing plenty of vitamins and nutrients... but there is even better news for slimmers.

Scientists have found that phytonutrients in raspberries can help to boost the rate at which fat is metabolized – have you seen all the raspberry ketone supplements that have taken the dieting industry by storm?

Have some - fresh, low-calorie and delicious.

Wash it down with a glass of orange juice to send your vitamin C levels sky-high.

Ingredients

- 1 oz unsweetened muesli
- 1 tbsp fat-free natural yogurt
- A handful of raspberries
- PLUS 1 glass unsweetened orange juice, ideally freshly squeezed

Method

1. Choose your favorite bowl and pour in the muesli – remember, do not add sugar or honey.

2. Top the muesli with the tablespoon of yogurt and the raspberries. Enjoy your fruity bowl along with your glass of orange juice.

Tomato Toast

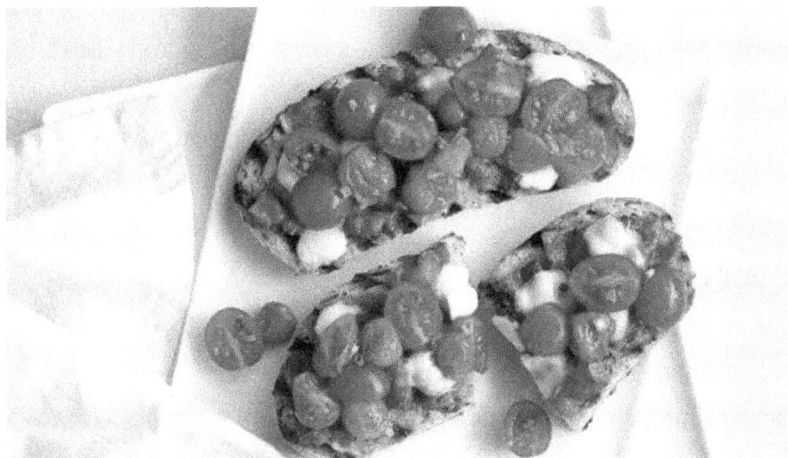

This quick and easy breakfast recipe is super-tasty and as healthy as anything, so enjoy it without guilt!

Bread can be controversial among dieters, but as long as it is a good quality whole-meal variety, it will be perfect for this 7-day plan.

We firmly believe in the nutritious power of high-fiber whole grains, but they do contain starch to do make sure you stick to just one slice, not three!

Tomatoes are an everyday superfood.

They are so good for us, but we sometimes take them for granted. Ripe tomatoes deliver a wonderful flavor and are bursting with lycopene.

Lycopene has been found to help prevent certain cancers, as well as diabetes and heart disease. It can also boost male fertility, support your eyesight, prevent skin aging and protect it from sun damage, plus it helps to prevent osteoporosis.

This unfussy recipe shows tomatoes off to their tasty best.

For the glass of juice, try freshly squeezing your own OJ, or if you have a juicer, try fresh pineapple.

Ingredients

- 1 slice of whole meal bread
- 3 cherry tomatoes
- Freshly ground black pepper (optional)
- PLUS 1 glass unsweetened fruit juice.

Method

1. Lightly toast the whole meal bread in the toaster on the lowest setting.

2. Meanwhile, slice the cherry tomatoes and pre-heat the grill to a medium heat.

3. Take the toast and arrange the cherry tomato slices on top. Place under the grill for 5 minutes, or until the tomatoes have softened and the toast has browned.

4. Remove and eat hot, with a grinding of black pepper, if you wish.

Poacher's Breakfast

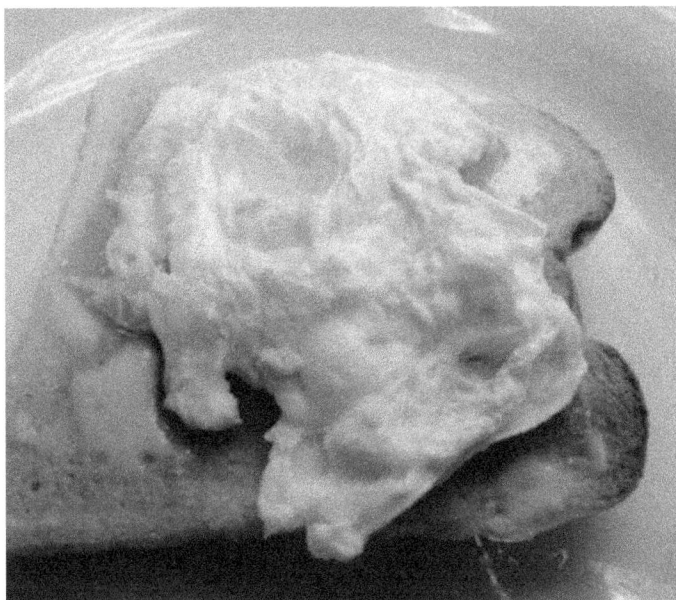

Eggs are a natural, delicious, superfood. Low-calorie and ultra-versatile, they are also protein-packed and highly nutritious – every serious dieter should stock up on plenty of the organic, free-range variety.

Nutrients include Vitamins A, B2, B5, B12, B6, D, E and K, plus folate, selenium, calcium and zinc – just fabulous!

Ingredients

- 2 small free-range eggs
- 1 slice of whole meal bread
- 1 drop of vinegar
- 1 pinch of salt (for the water only)

Method

1. First, get the eggs poaching. Put on a medium-sized saucepan of water to boil and add a pinch of salt to it. Make sure your egg is really fresh and crack one into a ramekin or cup. Add a small drop of vinegar to your egg.

2. When the water is boiling, take a hand-held balloon whisk and stir the water to create a gentle whirlpool in the water, which will help the egg white wrap around the yolk.

3. Slowly tip the egg into the water, white first. Turn the heat right down to the minimum setting. Leave to cook for three minutes.

4. Meanwhile, after about a minute and a half has passed, pop your whole meal bread in the toaster, so it should be ready at about the same time as your egg.

5. After three minutes, remove the egg with a slotted spoon, snipping off any straggly edges using the edge of the spoon.

6. Rest the egg to drain onto kitchen paper for a few seconds – this is an important step as a waterlogged dish is unpleasant. Place the egg onto the whole meal toast – no butter – and enjoy it hot.

Tropinana Smoothie

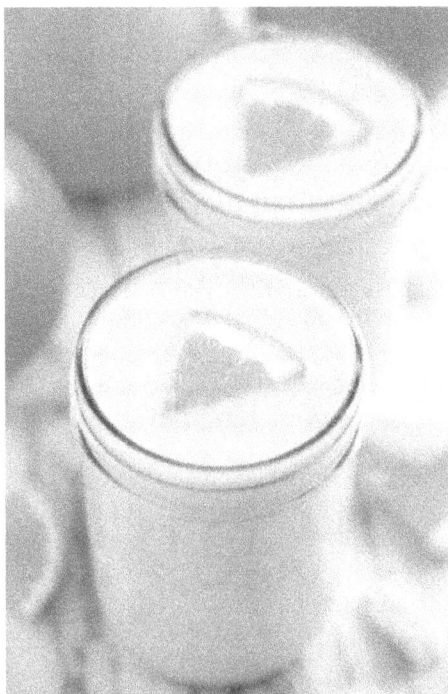

Sometimes you need a fruity start to the day... try this delicious smoothie, which will give you a fantastic dose of vitamin C from the orange, potassium from the banana and plenty of calcium too along with a host of other nutrients.

Plus, this tropical concoction tastes out of this world – a real sweet treat that makes a brilliant breakfast on any day.

Ingredients

- 1 large orange
- 1 banana
- 1/4pt semi-skimmed milk

- 1 small pot of natural yogurt
- 1tsp clear honey

Method

1. Peel the orange to remove all skin and pith and peel the banana, then chop them into pieces.

2. Place the fruit in a blender and pour in the milk and yogurt.

3. Whizz it all up in your blender and serve.

New York Summer

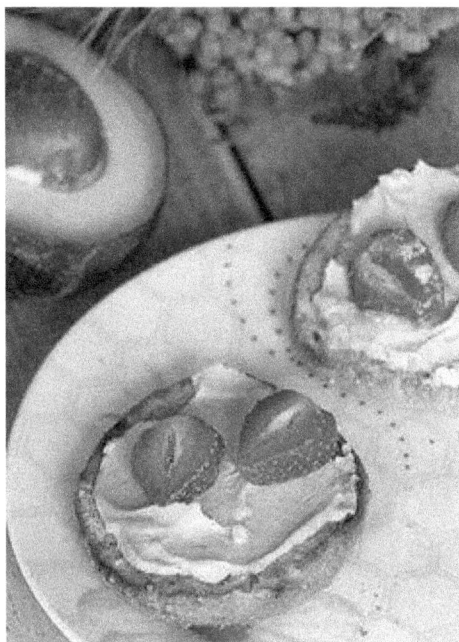

This delicious breakfast is fresh-tasting with the light, creamy cheese and juicy strawberries. The whole-wheat butter-free bagel will provide you with plenty of fiber.

Meanwhile, the delectable cream cheese packs a great calcium punch without the usual calories.

Finally, the strawberries are a total superfood – they are packed with antioxidant vitamin C, which boosts immunity, supports your eyesight, helps to combat cancer, stimulates collagen production and much more.

Plus, they are very low in calories and high in fiber.

So, as you can see, while this breakfast treat looks and feels somewhat naughty and decadent, it is extremely good for you, so don't hold back!

Ingredients

- 1 whole-wheat bagel
- 1tsp reduced-fat cream cheese
- A large handful of strawberries

Method

1. Slice the bagel into two halves and toast them.

2. When it is ready, spread the reduced fat cream cheese onto the hot bagel halves.

3. Eat hot, nibbling the strawberries alongside as a sweet treat.

Egg and Hummus Breakfast Wrap

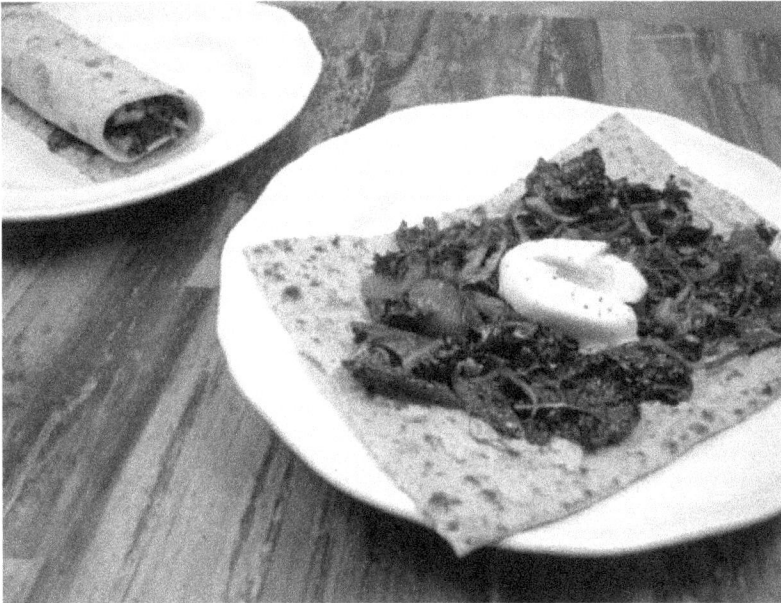

Time for a really wholesome and filling breakfast recipe. This is no ordinary wrap – it is bursting with the protein-packed goodness of eggs and chickpeas, plus nutrient-rich mushrooms and onions for a real hit of savory flavor and tasty textures.

The spinach is also a star of this dish – it is a powerful source of both iron and Vitamin C and it cleanses the blood – a great detoxifying leaf.

Ingredients

- 1 whole grain tortilla
- 1-2 tbsp hummus
- 1 large egg
- 1/4 cup egg whites

- 1/8 cup chopped onion
- 2 button mushrooms, sliced
- 2 cups baby spinach
- 1 tbsp crumbled reduced-fat feta
- 1 tbsp chopped sun-dried tomatoes
- Low-calorie cooking spray
- Freshly ground pepper, to taste (optional)
- Hot sauce (optional)

Method

1. Spray the skillet with the low-calorie cooking spray and sauté the onion and mushrooms for 3-4 minutes or until tender and fragrant.

2. Add spinach and sauté the vegetables for a few minutes longer, until spinach has wilted.

3. Add egg and egg whites to pan with veggies and cook for about 2 minutes or until eggs are cooked through. Add a grind of black pepper if you wish. Warm up the tortilla in the oven for a few minutes.

4. Spread a layer of hummus on the tortilla when ready. Place the eggs in the center of the tortilla and top with the sun-dried tomatoes and low-fat feta.

5. Season with more pepper as well as hot sauce if it takes your fancy. Wrap the tortilla up and serve!

Veggie Breakfast Bake

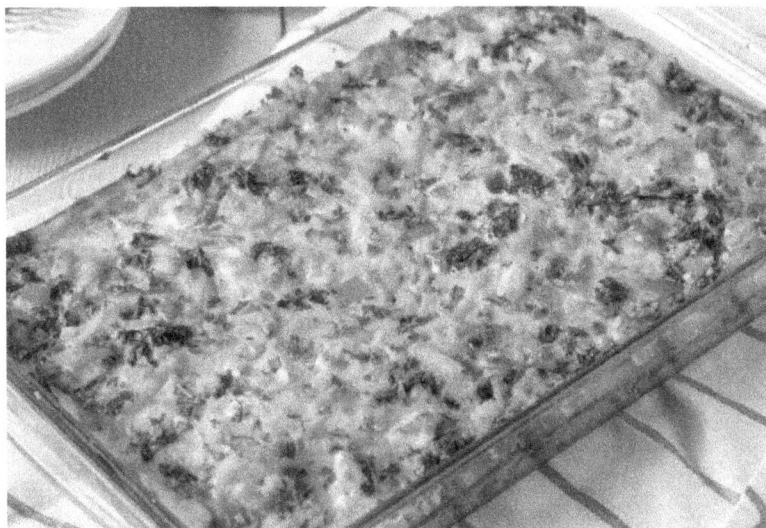

This is the last breakfast of the week, if you select them in order, so it could well take the place of a Sunday fry-up.

It is a totally delicious take on a cooked breakfast, with none of the fatty, processed bacon to ladle on the calories. It features the 'everyday superfood' tomatoes, plus powerfully iron-rich spinach and a lovely, large mushroom too.

Mushrooms have very few calories and have the added benefit of having been shown in studies to enhance weight loss.

Ingredients

- 1 large egg
- 1 large field mushroom
- 2 tomatoes, halved

- A large handful of spinach
- 1/2 garlic clove, thinly sliced
- 1 tsp olive oil

Method

1. Heat oven to 200C/180C fan/gas 6. Put the mushroom, tomatoes and slices of garlic into an ovenproof dish.

2. Drizzle over the oil and grind over pepper, then bake for 10mins.

3. Meanwhile, put the spinach into a colander, then pour over a kettle of boiling water to wilt it. Squeeze out any excess water, then add the spinach to the dish.

4. Make a little gap between the vegetables and crack an egg into each dish.

5. Return to the oven and cook for a further 8-10mins or until the egg is cooked to your liking.

If you feel like sharing the love and helping other readers decide if this is the right book for them, please take a few seconds to leave a short review on Amazon.com.

Chapter 7

Lunch Recipes

Welcome to your lovely lunch section – your choice of deliciously healthy mid-day meals. The recipes include a wide range of flavors and textures so there is no danger of getting bored – it's not all lettuce 24/7.

The selection of dished is varied but simple. There is certainly something here that you will enjoy and we hope that you love all 7 dishes on offer. The lunches will give you plenty of slow-burning and healthy energy, plus a kaleidoscope of colorful, flavorful nutrients all for remarkably few calories – the perfect recipe for success when you are aiming to lose weight.

In this chapter, the recipes offer plenty of healthy fiber, in a variety of forms, plus some tasty lean protein. All of the recipes opt for the healthier forms of carbohydrate, so you will be well fueled, but also nourished to just the right degree.

You won't feel hungry and stressed-out on this diet – just stick to the plan and enjoy some great food as you Drop A Dress Size in 7 Days. It is essential that you enjoy a good lunch every day. Regular good food will keep your energy levels up, which is vital for when you are exercising most days.

Plus, it will keep your metabolism revved up and burning faster, which is very important for when you want to keep the pounds dropping off.

Finally, it will help to keep your spirits high throughout the week, which will only make your diet more effective.

If you are the kind of person who grabs a quick bite on the go at lunchtime and sometimes falls into bad habit by choosing a greasy snack over something light, bright-tasting, properly nourishing and uplifting, then you are in for a real treat.

Also, of course you may not want to cook a full-on lunch every day, especially if you are working. So, these recipes are simple and light, without skimping on flavor or interest. The majority of them can be made in advance and stored for whenever you need them, or taken to work in a lunchbox, or heated up at the office.

When you are devoting your week to shedding the excess weight, then you don't need added complications, just delicious, easy to prepare meals.

Also, do remember that since these lunch recipes are mostly quite high in fiber, you may feel that you are eating more food than usual.

This is not the case in weight loss terms – fiber is your friend. It fills you up and helps to look after the digestive system. In fact, you will simply be enjoying, healthy, balanced meals with just a fraction of the calories.

So, get stuck in – every recipe here tastes wonderful!

Tricolore Salad

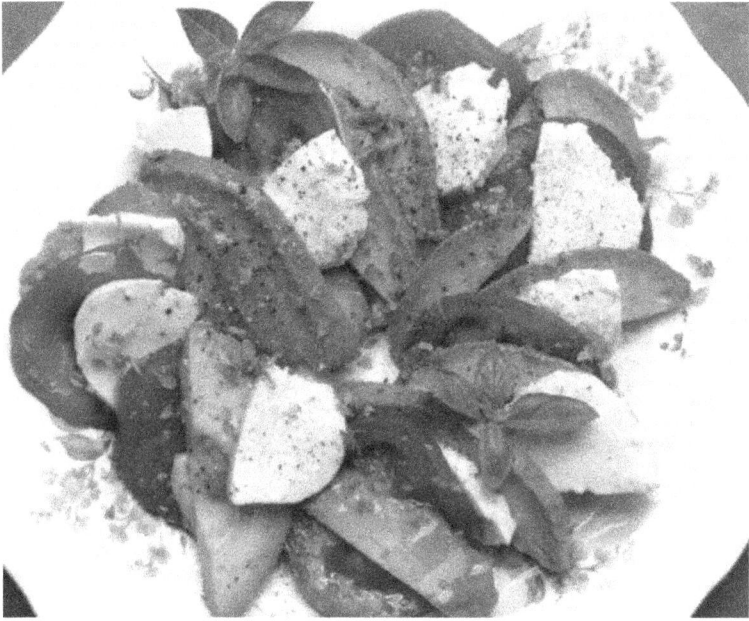

This "three-color" Italian salad may make you do a double-take at first, because it may appear to stray from the low-fat ethos.

The great news is that while it has some fat, these are the best types of fat for your health and they may even help you to lose weight.

Fresh-tasting, creamy avocados are a real nutritionists' favorite, being full of healthy fats.

Twinned with lycopene-rich tomatoes and calcium-packed mozzarella, it helps to make a truly delicious salad, with some crunchy wholegrain crackers on the side.

Ingredients

- 1 small avocado
- 1 tomato
- 2 oz reduced-fat mozzarella
- 2 wholegrain crackers

For the oil-free dressing

- 1 tbsp balsamic vinegar
- 1 tsp wholegrain mustard

Method

1. Slice up the tomato, avocado and reduced-fat mozzarella.

2. Mix the balsamic with the mustard, beating with a fork to thoroughly blend. Drizzle the oil-free dressing, over the salad.

3. Serve your Tricolore Salad and enjoy it with the two wholegrain crackers.

Your Choice Veggie Soup

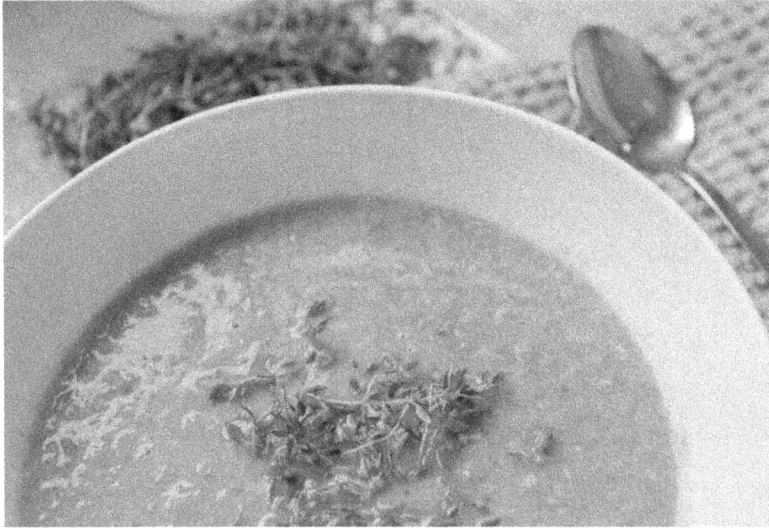

This lunch is great for when you want something warming and wholesome.

We call it "your choice" because it is one recipe where, if you fancy, you can take an easy shortcut. If you are pressed for time, or are working during the day, you may want to simply buy a soup.

If this is the case, go for a ready-made soup that is high in green veg like kale, not too heavy on the potato and is ideally free from additives and preservatives.

If in doubt and if you have enough time, the better option would be to make your down delicious vegetable soup from scratch. Just follow the simply recipe below.

Ingredients

For the Homemade Green Veg Soup

- 7oz zucchini, roughly sliced
- 2oz broccoli
- 4oz kale, chopped
- 500ml stock, made by mixing 1 tbsp bouillon powder and boiling water in a jug
- 2 garlic cloves, sliced
- A thumb-sized piece ginger, sliced
- ½ tsp ground coriander
- Thumb-sized piece fresh turmeric root, peeled and grated, or ½ tsp ground turmeric
- A pinch of kosher salt
- 1 lime, zested and juiced
- A bunch of parsley, roughly chopped, reserving some to serve
- 1 tbsp sunflower oil
- Plus, a whole-meal roll, to serve

Method

1. Put the oil in a deep pan, add the garlic, ginger, coriander, turmeric and salt, fry on a medium heat for 2 mins, then add 3 tbsp water to give a bit more moisture to the spices.

2. Add the zucchini, making sure you mix well to coat the slices in all the spices, and continue cooking for 3 mins.

3. Add 400ml stock and leave to simmer for 3 mins.

4. Add the broccoli, kale and limejuice with the rest of the stock. Leave to cook again for another 3-4 mins until all the vegetables are soft.

5. Take off the heat and add the chopped parsley. Pour everything into a blender and blend on high speed until it is a lovely smooth green with speckles of kale.

6. Garnish with lime zest and the reserved parsley, then serve, with a whole-meal roll on the side.

Garden Open Sandwich

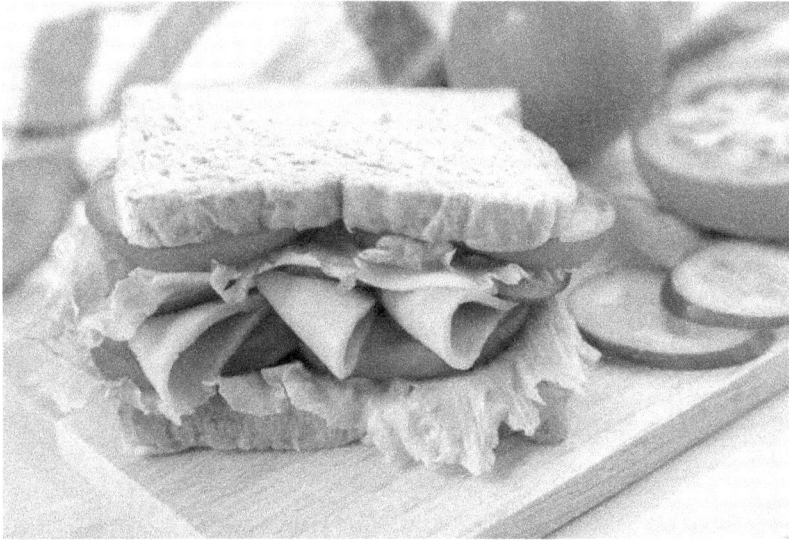

Sometimes you just want fast food. So, go for it! But happily, on this plan, that does not have to mean a fatty burger, quite the opposite.

When you want it fast and flavorsome, try this easy-to-make open sandwich which gives you everything you need in one delicious hit – lean protein in the ham, fiber and many other nutrients in the arugula and tomatoes, plus some wonderful whole-grain bread.

Sticking to one slice of whole-meal instead of two greatly lowers the calorie toll and creates a lighter, fresher dish.

You can even eat a calcium-rich, low-fat yogurt straight afterwards if you wish. Just make it quick, easy and totally enjoyable – the perfect workday lunch.

Ingredients

- 1 slice of whole-meal bread
- 2 slices of lean ham
- A handful of arugula leaves
- 2 tomatoes, sliced
- Plus 1 fat-free fruit yogurt for afterwards

Method

1. Lay the whole-meal bread on a plate. Top it with the ham, in ridges if possible for added texture.

2. Scatter over the arugula then top with the tomato slices. It's ready! Don't forget, you can enjoy a fat-free fruit yogurt afterwards if you fancy something sweet but light.

Piri-piri Prawn Pita

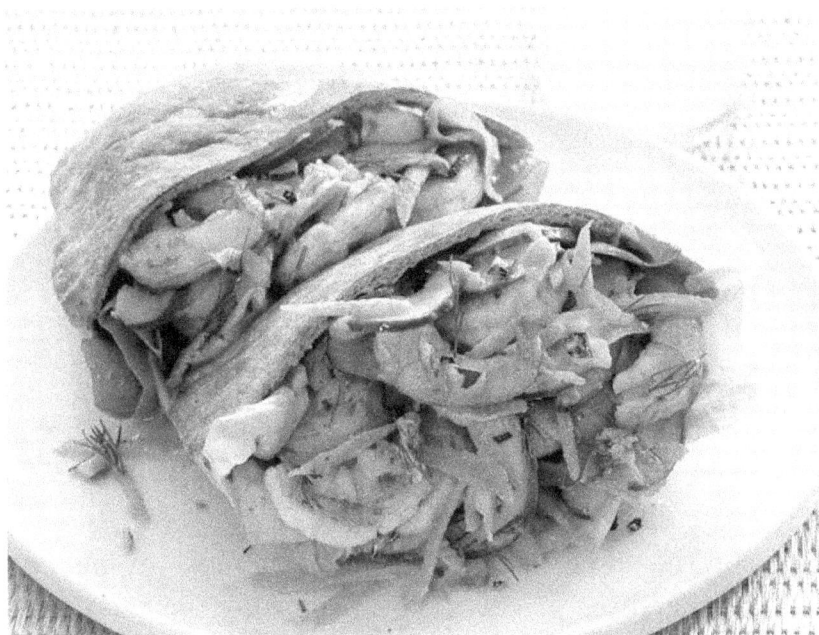

This is a super flavorsome pita lunch. Prawn are delicious, especially when perked up with a spike of chili.

Chili pepper is fantastic for speeding up the metabolism, so don't hold back. It's the perfect partner to ingredients on the Drop A Dress in 7 Days diet.

Ingredients

- A large handful of peeled raw king prawns
- 1 small whole-wheat pita bread
- A few leaves of gem lettuce
- ½ red pepper, sliced
- 1 tbsp fat-free sour cream

- Juice of ½ a lemon
- A handful of mint, finely chopped
- 1 tsp olive oil
- 1 garlic clove, crushed
- ¼ bird's-eye chili, finely chopped (remove the seeds unless you want it very hot
- Sprinkling of paprika

Method

1. Heat oven to 160C/140C fan/gas 3. Mix the fat-free soured cream with a squeeze of lemon juice, the fresh mint and seasoning, cover and put in the fridge.

2. Put the oil in a skillet and heat it on medium-high. Add in the slices of red pepper and cook them until they start to soften.

3. Meanwhile, wrap the pita pocket in foil and heat it in the oven.

4. Add in the prawns to the skillet, another squeeze of lemon juice, the garlic, chili, paprika and seasoning. Cook and stir until the prawns are cooked through. Remove the heated pita and slice a slit into it. Place it on a plate.

5. Stuff the pita pocket with lettuce, plus the pepper and prawn mixture. Top with the cold, seasoned fat-free soured cream and enjoy.

Cheesy Jacket

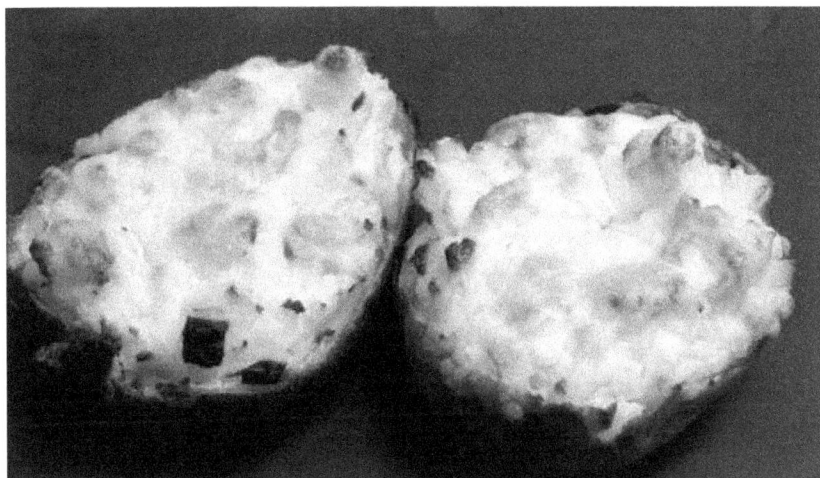

Sometimes there is nothing better than the simple things in life. A good, fiber-rich baked potato makes a delicious lunch.

Follow it up with a refreshing sunshine burst of orange, dripping with vitamin C, and you are all set to enjoy an active afternoon.

Ingredients

- 1 jacket potato, no bigger than your fist
- 2 tbsp low-fat cottage cheese
- Plus, 1 orange for afterwards

Method

1. Pre-heat the oven to 350°F.

2. Stab the potato several times with a sharp knife, so that it cooks right through. It may take around an hour. TIP – it you are short for time, soften the potato first in a microwave by placing on high for 10 minutes.

3. When the skin of the potato is crispy and browned, then remove. Cut the potato nearly in half and top with the low-fat cottage cheese. Ready to serve this dish, which is high in fiber and high on satisfaction. Enjoy an all-natural dessert of orange segments.

Bean Crunch

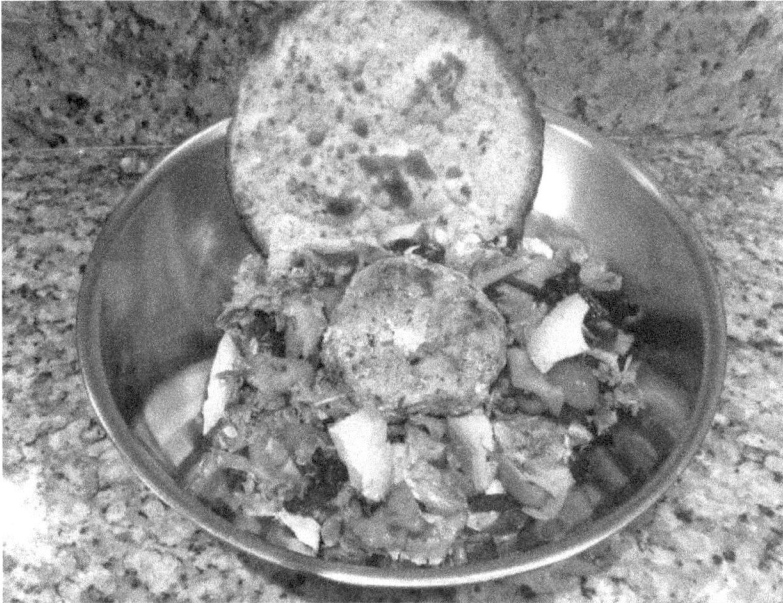

This is a tasty dish with a difference. Bean salad is delicious and filling, but high-protein pulses tend to get left off the menu far too often.

This easy to prepare dish is simple and straightforward, marrying the rich textures and flavors of beans with creamy hummus and crispy, crunchy rice cakes.

This recipe, once again, has two parts. If you are crazy busy, you can simply go to a deli near your office and take away 4oz of bean salad.

However, you are taking a bit of a risk as it may be too heavy in terms of added olive oil, or even additives.

Why not take an extra 5 minutes and play it safe by making our delicious bean salad yourself?

You are guaranteed bags of low-calorie flavor and can control the levels of fat. The recipe below makes more than you will need for one meal, but it keeps for days and tastes even better after a short spell in the fridge.

Ingredients

- 4oz quick homemade bean salad
- 2 rice cakes, topped
- Low-fat hummus
- Plus 1 apple

To make the bean salad

- 1 x 14 oz (400g) can of organic mixed beans
- 1 small onion, finely chopped
- 3 tbsp white wine vinegar
- ½ tbsp light olive oil
- A handful or flat-leaf parsley, finely chopped

Method

1. Drain the can of beans and pour them into a medium bowl.

2. Add the onions to the beans and mix.

3. In another bowl, mix the white wine vinegar and the olive oil, whipping with a fork to form a light vinaigrette emulsion.

4. Scatter the chopped parsley over the beans and onions, then pour over the vinaigrette.

5. Season to taste and mix well with a fork, then, if you have time, let the salad sit for at least 10 minutes to deepen the flavors.

To make the Bean Crunch

1. Lay the rice cakes on a plate and spread them thinly with low-fat hummus.

2. Top the rice cakes with bean salad – pile them high, it's all good! Enjoy with a large glass of water and the apple for afterwards.

Tasty Turkey Wrap

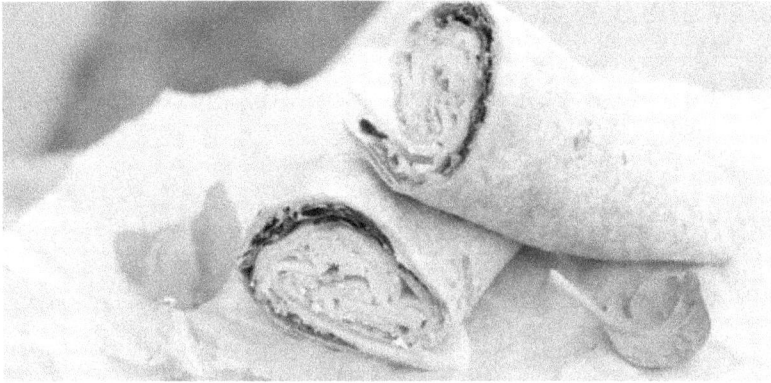

Turkey is a delicious source of lean protein that all too often gets forgotten until the holiday season.

Make the most of the protein-packed goodness in this superb light lunch which brings together calcium-rich goat cheese, iron-rich spinach, plus all the protein, folate and weight-loss enhancing fiber in hummus.

So many good flavors and textures, it makes for the perfect weekday lunch.

Ingredients

- 1 whole-wheat wrap
- 3 slices deli turkey
- 2 tablespoons hummus
- 1 tablespoon low-fat goat cheese
- 1 handful baby spinach

Method

1. Warm the whole wheat wrap (optional).

2. Spread the wrap with the hummus, lay over with turkey slices.

3. Top with goat cheese and scatter over the baby spinach. Eat warm.

Chapter 8

Dinner Recipes

A delicious dinner is a wonderful thing and just because you may be on a weight loss plan, there is absolutely no reason why you can't fully enjoy it!

A week is not long, but far too long to eat dull, tasteless dinners.

At the same time, after a busy day we do not all want to be cooking for hours, especially when we don't want to be thinking about food all the time – dinner should be simple, nutritious and enjoyable.

These dinners get the balance just right.

This chapter will tell you how to prepare dinners that offer a range of different and interesting flavors.

There are plenty of vegetables and some lean protein, alongside light portions of carbohydrates – all the elements of a great healthy supper.

One important piece of advice should be heeded though when it comes to dinner. Do try not to eat late at night, ideally not after 7pm.

After this time, the body slows down and prepares for the night sleep. When you go to sleep, your meal may not be fully digested and the food sits there, plus your sluggish body take the cue to start laying down reserves of fat instead of burning of the food through exercise, for example.

Late-night eating will not help your cause, so if you tend to eat a late dinner, try bringing it forward to earlier in the evening – the habit may hopefully stick beyond 7 days.

You are likely to want to try all 7 dinner recipes on offer, but do not feel tied to it – you are free to repeat your favorites during the week if you like.

However, if you do enjoy all 7 dinners during the week, you will benefit from a great variety of essential nutrients.

Plus remember, they are all wonderfully low in calories and fat, so tuck in without guilt and look forward to losing even more weight as you go!

Lemon Salmon

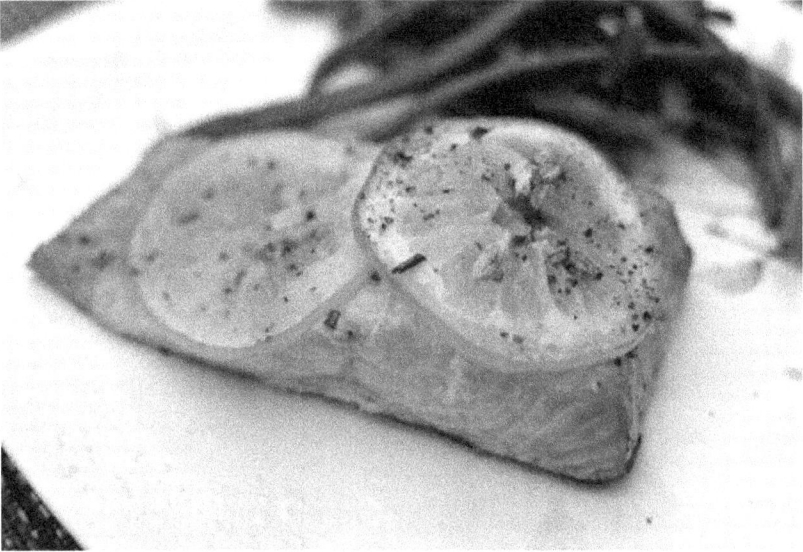

Salmon is a delicious oily fish that nutritionists love, thanks to its richness in omega-3 essential fatty acids.

The delicious pink flesh is low calorie and goes beautifully with a burst of fresh, Vitamin C-packed lemon.

The vegetables offer every possible combination of vitamins and minerals, depending on which you choose.

Try a few of these, chopped into bite-sized pieces – broccoli, peppers, carrots, spring onions, mushrooms... or any vegetable you fancy that is not too starchy.

Cook them to the degree of doneness you like, but leaving them on the crunchy side will help retain their nutrients.

Ingredients

- 1 medium salmon fillet
- Juice of 1 lemon
- 3 1/2oz mixed vegetables
- 1tsp olive oil

Method

1. Preheat the oven to 180°C. Squeeze lemon over the salmon and wrap it in foil, then bake it for about 12mins.

2. As it cooks, take a small wok or skillet and stir-fry the vegetables in the olive oil. When both the salmon and the vegetables are ready, serve and enjoy.

Tomato and Herb Chicken

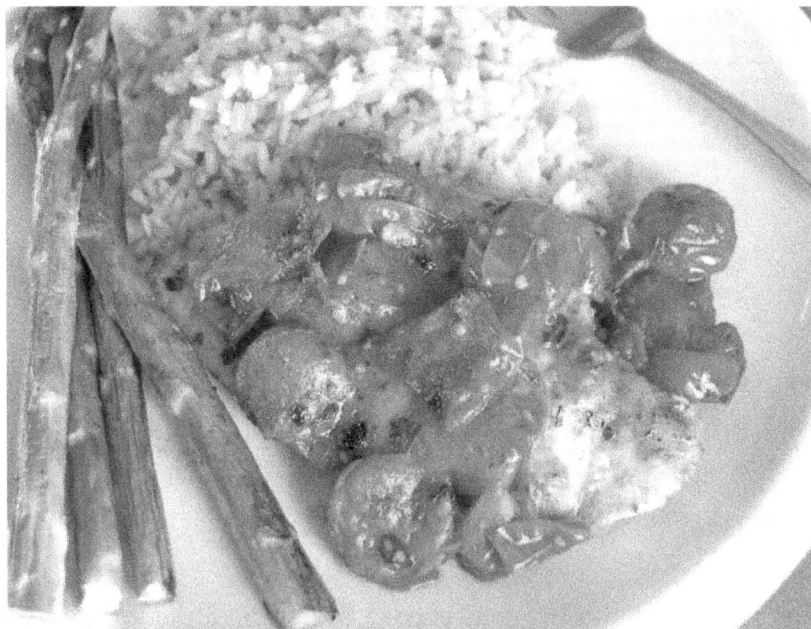

The delicious lean protein of chicken goes perfectly with the fruity goodness of tomatoes in this dish. The broccoli is ultra-low in calories, but full of fiber and nutrients.

The carrots are fabulous too, sweet in taste and also full of fiber, plus carotene, which helps to ward off a wide range of diseases including heart disease.

The vegetables are full of vitamins, which will support you as you lose weight and the steaming will retain more nutrients than boiling.

Warming and earthy, this dish will fill you up nicely and is deceptively low in calories.

Also, don't forget you can enjoy a couple of delicious plums afterwards - they are rich in bone-healthy Vitamin K and taste great too.

Ingredients

- 1 chicken fillet
- A small tin of plum tomatoes
- 2 tsp mixed dried herbs
- 2 ¼ oz broccoli
- 2 ¼ oz carrots
- Plus, 2 plums for dessert.

Method

1. Pre-heat the oven to 190°C. Place the chicken breast in an ovenproof dish.

2. Break up the plum tomatoes a little with a fork and pour them over the chicken.

3. Sprinkle over the dried herbs, mixing them in a little with the fork. Place the chicken and tomato dish in the oven and cook for 15-20mins.

4. When the chicken is nearly ready, cut the broccoli into florets and chop the carrot then steam over boiling water in a colander, or in a special steamer, if you have one.

5. Ensure the chicken is cooked through with no pink and serve it in the sauce with the vegetables, when they are tender.

Sausages and Sweet Potato Mash

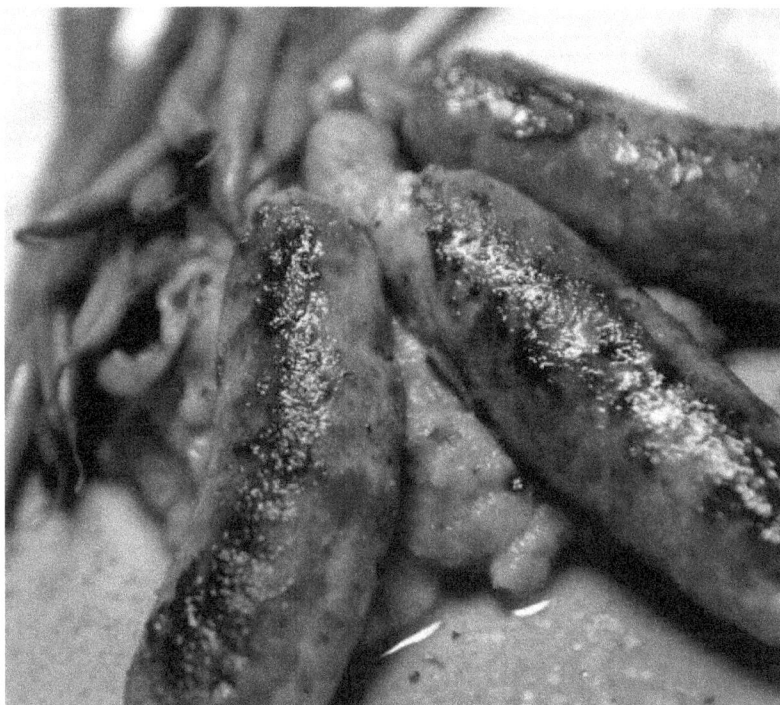

Sausages, on a diet? Yes, sure!

This lovely dish combines the best type of comfort food with bags of flavor and it will all help you lose weight too – a great win-win!

The sausages to use in this dish are the best quality lean beef sausages that you can find. This will keep the fat levels down to a minimum, without reducing taste. Sweet potato is a healthier option for slimmers than normal white potato. It is higher in fiber and lower in calories and carbohydrates, so it makes a great choice.

Even the crème fraiche, which makes the sweet potato mash feel silky and luxurious, is another calcium-rich, low-fat version.

Ingredients

- 2 lean beef sausages
- 4oz green beans
- 1oz sweet potato
- 1tsp low-fat crème fraiche

Method

1. Preheat the grill to a medium high heat and place the sausages under it to cook, turning occasionally for 15-20 minutes.

2. Cut the sweet potato into cubes and place in a pan of water to boil for 15 minutes or until tender.

3. When the sausages and sweet potato are nearly ready, wither place a small colander over the boiling water, place the green beans in and steam for 3 or 4 minutes, or use a steamer until they are just tender.

4. Drain the sweet potato and mash in the pan using a potato masher. Stir the teaspoon of crème fraiche into the sweet potato.

5. Serve the sausages, with the scoop of sweet potato mash and the green beans while still hot.

Lamb Chop with Summer Veg

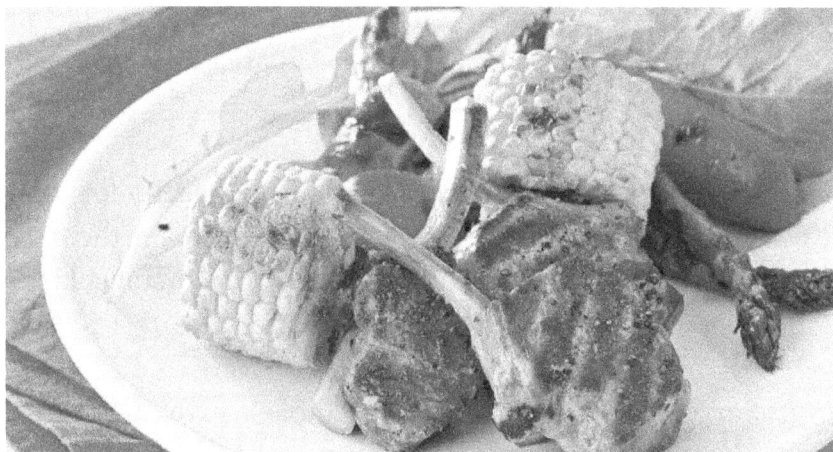

Lamb is a delicious red meat that you may have thought was "off-limits" as you drop a dress size in 7 Days.

Some people find it to be fatty meat, but this depends on the way you prepare it – it certainly doesn't have to be.

Happily, we know how to cook is so it remains low in fat and calories and high in protein – grilled, with as little fat as possible. Just steam some sugar snap peas, for plenty of vitamin K, A and folic acid, plus corn and serve alongside the lamb for a simple, flavorful dish.

Ingredients

- 1 small lamb chop
- 2 ¼ oz sugar snap peas
- 2 ¼ oz corn

Method

1. Trim the lamb of any excess fat if your butcher has not done this for you. It will still taste great and your body will thank you for it!

2. Place the chop under a medium-high grill for 10-12 minutes or until done to your liking. Steam the sugar snap peas and sweet corn by placing in a metal colander over a pan of boiling water for 3-4 minutes.

3. Serve the hot chop and vegetables, with just a little black pepper to taste if you fancy.

Chicken Stir-Fry with Noodles

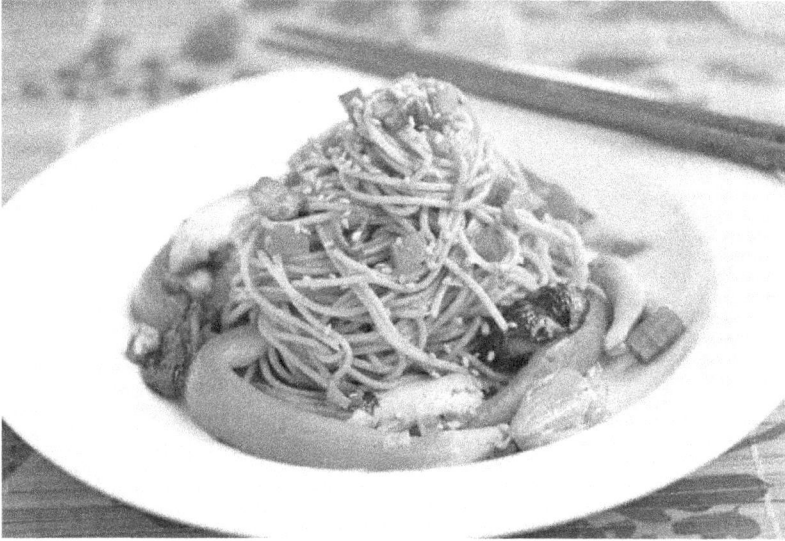

Chicken is a regular, high protein, low-fat slimmer's favorite but don't feel that you have to have it just plain grilled. This tasty stir fry packs so much color and flavor onto your plate that you'll love filling up on all these nutrients.

As a tasty, filling treat, this stir-fry is served with some delicious egg noodles for that authentic oriental taste.

Ingredients

- 1 chicken breast (no skin), cut into strips
- 4 mushrooms, sliced
- 3 cherry tomatoes, sliced in two
- A handful of sugar snap peas, sliced
- A handful of baby spinach
- 2oz of egg noodles

- 1tbsp oil

Method

1. Bring a small pan of water to the boil. When boiling, drop in the egg noodles and cook for 3-5 minutes, or until just tender. Drain and set aside.

2. Heat the oil in a wok or large skillet. When the oil is really hot, add the sliced chicken to the wok. Fry for 5-7 minutes, stirring and turning with a wooden spatula.

3. When the chicken is nearly cooked (if in doubt, test with a knife to ensure no pink is showing), add the sliced vegetables but not the spinach to the wok, stirring as they cook for 2-3 minutes.

4. Before the vegetables start to go too soft – they should retain a little 'bite' - add the cooked noodles and spinach to the wok.

5. Turn down the heat and stir the ingredients around together for 1-2 minutes until the spinach has wilted and the noodles have picked up the flavors and warmed through again. Remove the stir-fry into a bowl and serve piping hot.

Mediterranean Cod with Wedges

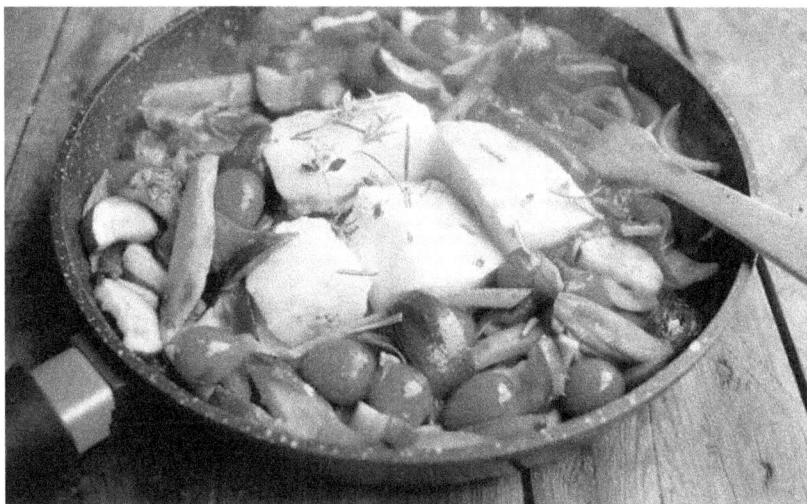

Cod is a wonderful fish. In fact, it has famously proven so popular over the years that the availability of stocks has been called into question, but happily much has been done to assure more sustainable cod is available, so buy some good quality cod to enjoy whenever you wish.

It is a primary source of super-lean protein, vitamin B12, iodine and selenium plus many more nutrients.

This particular dish is very tasty, thanks to the tomato-based sauce and crispy, lower-carb sweet potato wedges.

The kale is an excellent addition to your plate - full of calcium, antioxidants and super-healthy, purifying compounds, so don't miss out, it will help weight come off!

Ingredients

- 1 chunky cod fillet (or another white flaky fish, such as Pollack)
- 1 onion, chopped
- 400g can chopped tomatoes
- A few sprigs thyme, leaves stripped
- 3 oz kale, chopped
- ½ small sweet potato
- 1 tbsp low sodium soy sauce
- 1 tbsp olive oil

Method

1. Preheat the oven to 180°C. Peel the sweet potato and slice into finger-sized wedges. Drizzle lightly with half the olive oil and place on a baking tray. Put into the oven for 20 minutes.

2. Meanwhile, heat the remaining olive oil in a large skillet, add the onion, and then fry for 5-8 minutes until lightly browned.

3. Stir in the tomatoes, thyme and soy sauce, then bring it to the boil. Put a pan of water on to boil, ready for the kale.

4. Let the sauce simmer for 5 mins, then slip the cod into the skillet as well. Cover and gently cook for 8-10 mins until the cod flakes easily.

5. When the cod is ready, drop the kale into the boiling water and blanch it for several seconds. Drain in a colander and put on a plate.

6. Add the sweet potato wedges onto the plate with the kale, place the cod alongside and spoon over the warm tomato and onion sauce. Ready to eat and totally delectable!

Hot and Spicy Prawn Noodles

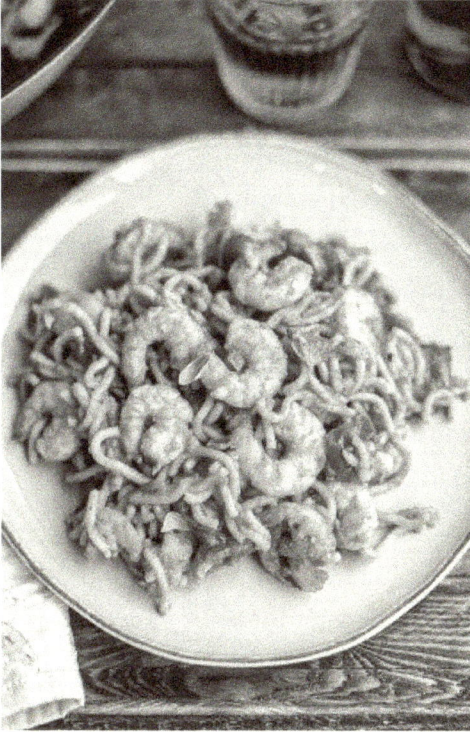

End your week (or begin it, as you prefer) with a totally flavor-packed and spicy dish.

This Chinese-inspired dish brings together a whole host of great, low-calorie foods, all served up in one bowl.

Prawns, which are a good source of protein and omega-3 fatty acids, lycopene-rich tomatoes, iron-rich spinach, all the vitamin C in the sweet juice and many more vitamins and nutrients besides in this low-fat dish.

Ingredients

- 2 oz egg noodles
- 4 oz cooked king prawns, defrosted if frozen
- ¼ large cucumber
- 2 scallions, finely sliced
- 6-8 cherry tomatoes, halved
- 1 green chili, deseeded, finely chopped
- 2 large handfuls of baby spinach leaves
- 4 tbsp low-calorie sweet chili sauce
- 1 low sodium vegetable bouillon cube
- Zest and juice of 1 lime
- 4/5 roasted cashews, crushed

Method

1. Boil a pan of water and add the vegetable bouillon cube and stir to make stock. Add the noodles to the boiling stock for 4 mins, then drain and set aside.

2. Warm the prawns in a small skillet for a minute or two, then turn off the heat.

3. Slice the cucumber lengthways into thick matchsticks. Add to the noodles with the scallions, tomatoes, chili and hot prawns.

4. In a small bowl, place the lime zest, juice and chili sauce and mix with a fork to make a dressing. Fold the dressing through the noodles.

5. Put a handful of spinach onto each serving plate, top with the prawn noodles sprinkle the crushed cashews over the top.

Others who are considering purchasing this book would love to know what you think. If you could spare a few seconds, they would greatly appreciate reading an honest review from you. Simply visit it on Amazon.com.

Chapter 9

Snack Options

So, we have run through all the great-tasting meals that you will be able to enjoy at breakfast, lunch and dinner. Now it is time to pick and choose what you fancy from the snack options available.

These snacks are all healthy, low-calorie and low in fat, just like the main meal. They are wholesome and full of helpful nutrients that will encourage your body to work at its best.

Plus, by enjoying a snack twice a day, remember – you will ensure that your metabolism works at its peak function.

That means burning calories even faster, so keep eating your snacks to keep losing weight!

Sounds great, right?

Well, it really is that simple – just follow the plan and you will certainly lose weight. All you have to do now is pick 2 favorite snacks each day from the following 14 suggestions.

Enjoy!

Cheesy Oatcakes

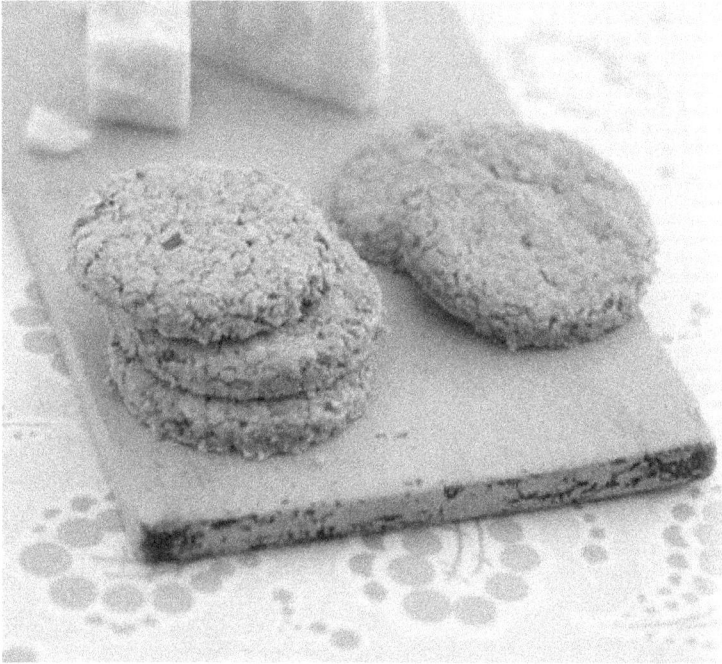

This is a quick, fun and surprisingly filling snack.

Oatcakes are a fantastic form of healthy-healthy, slow-burning carbs. They contain excellent fiber and leave you feeling fuller for longer. Traditionally partnered with cheese, this low-fat cottage cheese gives you taste without the calories.

Ingredients

- 3 organic oatcakes
- 2 tbsp reduced-fat cottage cheese
- 1 tsp chives, finely chopped (optional)

Method

1. Take the two oatcakes and lay them on a plate. Top each oatcake with 1 tablespoon of low-fat cottage cheese.

2. If you like, sprinkle the chopped chives over the cheese, then eat.

Crudités and Hummus

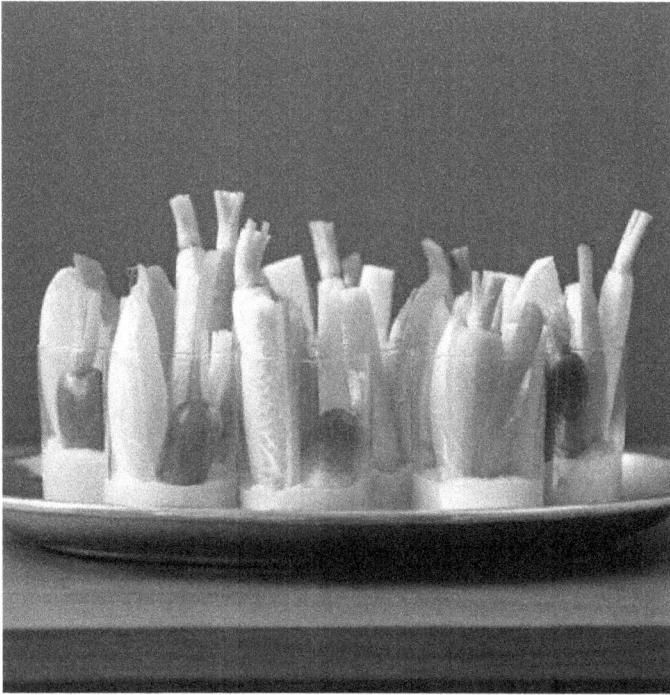

This is a great snack to tuck into when you are keen to eat something fresh-tasting and filling.

Raw vegetables are simply fantastic snacks; the best nature has to offer. They offer the highest levels of nutrients, as some gets lost when you cook your veg.

Add to them some creamy, chickpea-based hummus and you have a super snack that is worthy of the name.

Ingredients

- ½ cucumber

- 1 large carrot
- 2 sticks celery
- 8 radishes
- 1 tbsp reduced-fat hummus

Method

1. Chop the cucumber across in half, so you now have two quarters, the slice the quarters lengthways, so you end up with fat matchsticks of cucumber, about the thickness of a little finger.

2. Repeat with the carrot, chopping it into similar size matchsticks. Repeat as you chop the celery. Chop each radish in half.

3. Arrange all the vegetables on a large plate in their groups. Leave a good gap in the center. Into the gap spoon the tablespoon of reduced fat hummus.

4. To enjoy the crudités, simply pick a piece of veg and use the hummus as a healthy dip.

Quick Veggie Broth

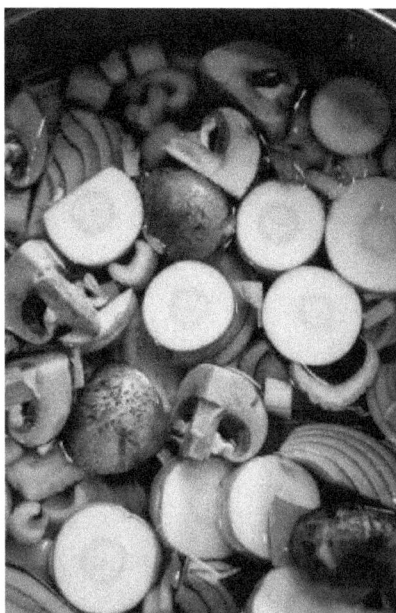

On a cold day, you might want a hot snack that will warm you up without piling on the calories, especially if you have had one of the light breakfast options.

Make this simple, light broth with a few vegetables. It basically just lots of fiber, water and nutrients, and it's really filling and delicious.

You can make larger amounts and store some in the fridge for another snack time or to reheat at the office.

Ingredients

- 1 cup water
- 1 large carrot

- 2 celery stalks
- 4 broccoli florets, chopped into small florets
- ½ onion
- 8 mushrooms, quartered
- 1 organic chicken stock cube
- 2 sprigs of fresh parsley

Method

1. Bring the water to the boil in a pan. Toss in an organic chicken stock cube, reduce to a simmer and stir until it dissolves.

2. Chop 1 large carrot, some broccoli florets, a few mushrooms and two celery stalks, then slice the onion into rings and add them to the stock.

3. Simmer for 5 minutes until the vegetables are tender and the stock has reduced a little, then remove to a bowl.

4. Season with pepper, tear the parsley and scatter it over the broth then, serve.

Crackerels

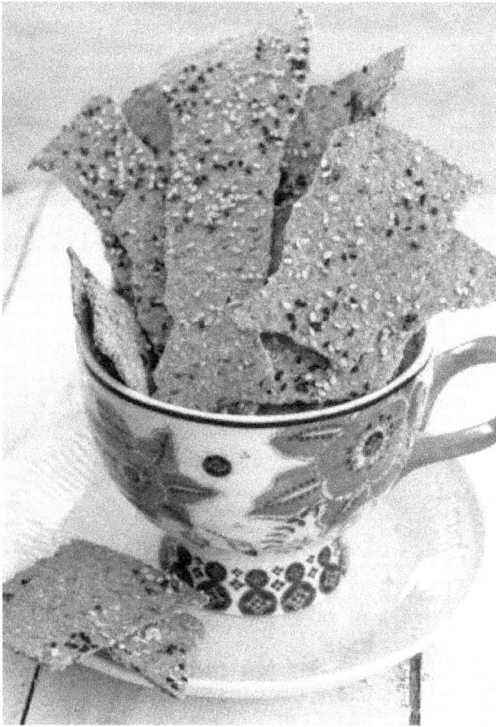

This is a fishy mid-afternoon treat, great for if you have just worked out or are planning a busy day.

Mackerel is an under-used oily fish that has super levels of essential fatty acids. It goes brilliantly with cracker and here it makes the basis of a lovely fish spread, the star of a mouth-watering snack.

Ingredients

- ½ small fillet of smoked mackerel
- 2 wholegrain crackers

- 1 tbsp fat-free plain yogurt
- 1 sprig parsley
- Freshly ground black pepper

Method

1. Remove any skin from the mackerel half-fillet and place it in bowl. Add the plain yogurt and mash it up the mackerel until it forms a coarse paste.

2. Lay the whole-grain cracker on a plate and top them with the healthy mackerel paté.

3. Chop up the parsley leaves and sprinkle over the cracker and paté. Finish off with a grinding of black pepper and enjoy.

Fruit Portion

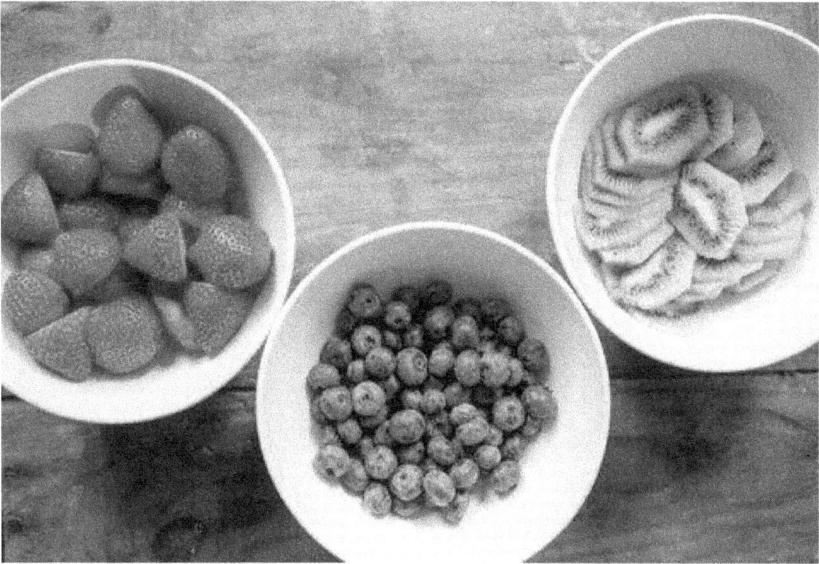

No recipe here exactly, just a hand list of good types and amounts of fruits to enjoy as a snack.

This is a handy quick comparison list, since a couple of grapes will not fill you up but a whole pineapple is definitely too much!

It will help you keep your calorie intake light since fruit, though delicious and healthy, does contain natural sugars, so you shouldn't fill up on it all day long and certainly not while on this plan.

Just pick a portion and enjoy it as your morning or afternoon snack.

Ingredients

- 1 apple
- 4 apricots
- 1 banana
- 1 cup mixed berries
- 1 cup blueberries
- 2 figs
- 1½ cups fresh fruit salad
- ½ grapefruit
- 12 grapes
- 1 guava
- 1 kiwi fruit
- ½ mango
- 1 cup melon
- 1 orange
- 4 passion fruit
- 1 cup pawpaw
- 1 peach
- 1 pear
- 4 rings pineapple
- 2 plums
- 3 prunes
- 2 satsumas
- 1½ cups strawberries
- 1 slice watermelon

Rye Crispbread 'Pizza'

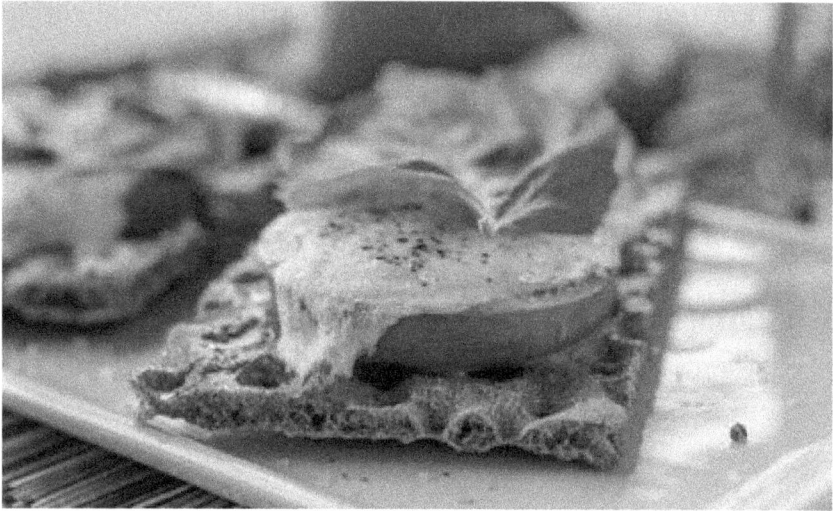

Rye crispbread are crunchy and wholesome alternatives to bread and just as versatile. They also make great snack, as is the case with this pizza-inspired low-calorie treat.

Even after you have completed the plan, you might like to enjoy the occasional pair of crispbreads topped with healthy, flavorsome foods like this as a far lighter alternative to a lunchtime sandwich at your desk – they travel well.

Ingredients

- 1 rye crispbread
- 1 medium ripe tomato
- 1 tbsp low-fat cottage cheese
- A few leaves of basil

Method

1. Lay out the rye crispbread. Top with the low-fat cottage cheese, spreading it right to the edges.

2. Slice the tomato into medium-thick circles and place them in a layer of over-lapping circles along the whole rye crispbread.

3. Roughly tear up the basil and scatter it over your snack, then eat.

Yogurt Snack

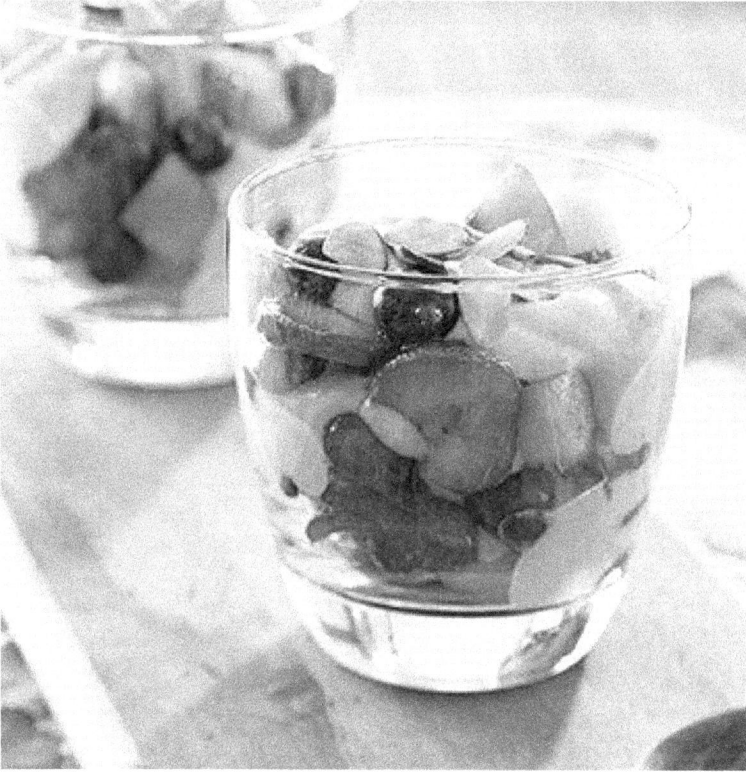

This is a fresh uncomplicated snack choice that requires no real preparation.

Yogurt is a superb food for dieters. Remember the study we discussed earlier in this book, where dieters who ate some yogurt daily lost more belly fat and retained more lean muscle than those who did not eat yogurt?

Great, then you will understand why this makes such a perfect snack.

Ingredients

- 150ml fat-free plain yogurt
- ½ from the list of fruit portion

Method

1. Chop your chosen fruit portion into small manageable pieces.

2. Stir into the yogurt. Serve chilled.

Apple Chips

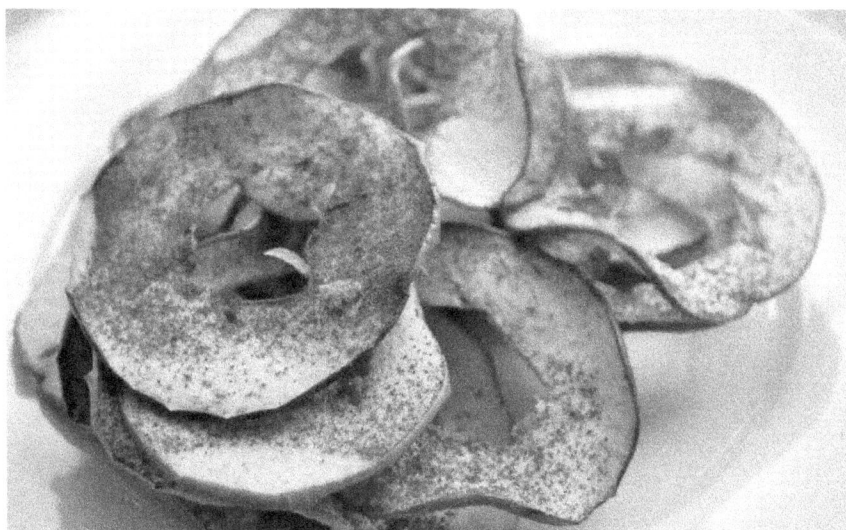

These apple chips can also be made in larger batches and stored in an airtight container for up to 3 days. They are good to take into work to enjoy when your energy levels dip during the afternoon.

Don't be tempted to add any sugar to this recipe, there is enough natural fructose to give a lovely sweet and sour taste, brought out by the cinnamon. Cinnamon lowers cholesterol and reduces inflammation so do add the whole teaspoonful!

Ingredients

- 2 red apples
- 1 tsp cinnamon

Method

1. Preheat the oven to 200 F. Thinly slice two apples crosswise about 1/8-inch (2 mm) thick with a mandolin or sharp knife.

2. Arrange apple slices in a single layer on baking sheets.

3. Sprinkle 1 teaspoon of cinnamon evenly over apple slices. Bake for 2 hours or until apples are dry and crisp, then eat.

Kale Smoothie

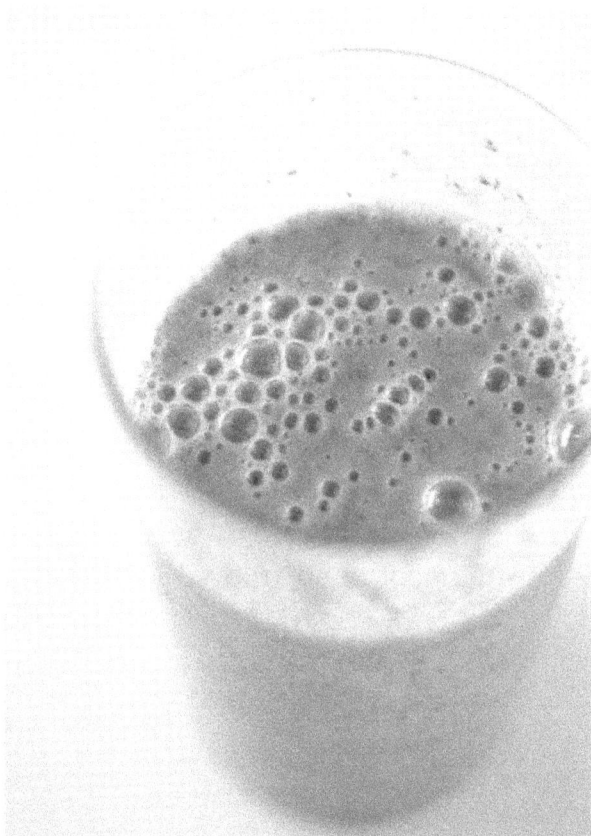

This smoothie features lots of kale, which is a dark green super-leaf. Kale is full of calcium, antioxidants and ultra-healthy, purifying compounds, which are all excellent news when you are trying to shed the toxins and the pounds.

Not everyone jumps at the idea of drink a green smoothie, but the taste is softened by the apple juice and banana. Drink this when you want a shot of liquid greens – there is nothing like it for a burst of helpful nutrients.

Ingredients

- ¾ cup chopped kale, ribs and thick stems removed
- 1 stalk celery, chopped
- ½ small banana
- ½ cup unsweetened apple juice
- 1 tablespoon fresh lemon juice
- ½ cup ice

Method

1. Place the kale, celery, banana, apple juice, ice, and lemon juice in a blender.

2. Blend until smooth and frothy then drink it nice and cold.

Popcorn Time

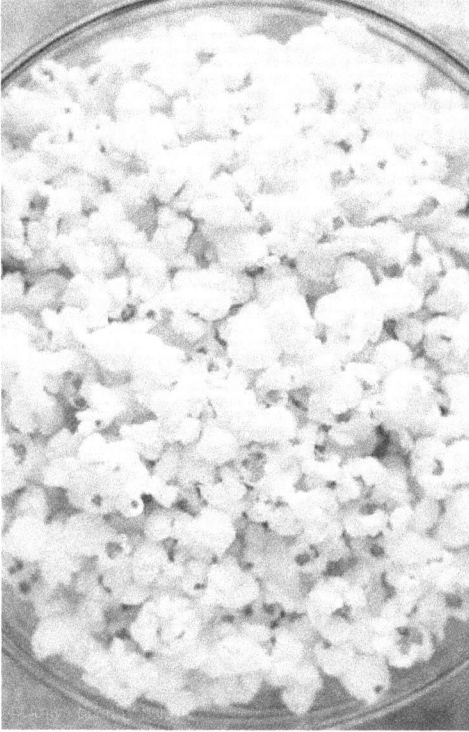

Most people are amazed when they learn how low in calories popcorn can be when it is made fresh at home.

It is a very good source of fiber, so will keep you feeling full for longer, making it a top snack. Also, it's super easy to make!

Ingredients

- 20g of popping corn (just 62kcal!)
- 1 tsp of oil

Method

1. Tip the oil into a medium-sized pan followed by the popping corn. Cover the pan with its lid – important!

2. Heat until you hear popping, or can see the corn jumping through a glass lid.

3. Keep the heat and lid on for 1-2 minutes until the popping slows right down to the odd burst. Listening is the key – you don't want burnt popcorn! Tip into a bowl and eat it warm. Wonderful.

Banana Milkshake

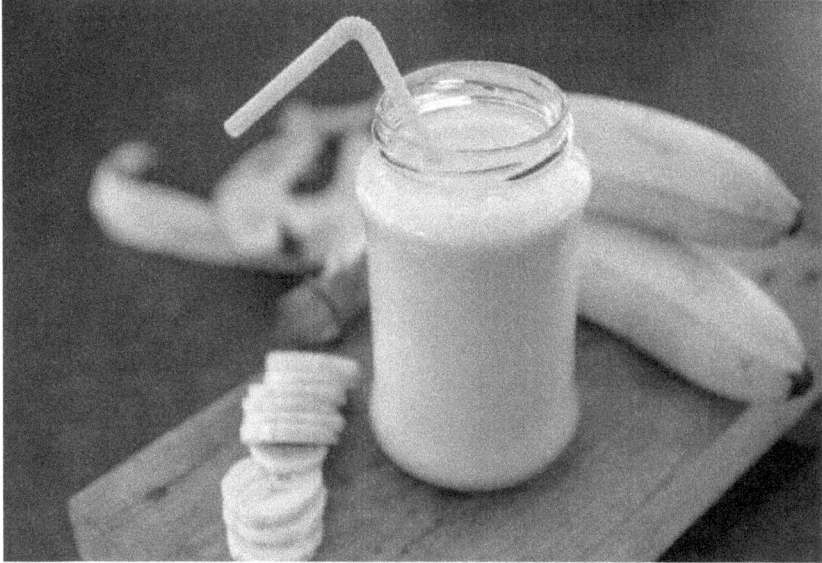

Sounds very indulgent and fattening – but of course this version certainly isn't! Milkshakes are such a childhood treat that they can be a hard habit to shake (excuse the pun). No need to worry though if you use skim milk or low-fat milk.

You can simply enjoy the smooth, soothing taste as you top up your calcium levels, plus the potassium from the banana. A snack that really hits the spot if you have a sweet craving.

Ingredients

- 100ml low-fat milk
- 1 very ripe banana
- Ground cinnamon (optional)

Method

1. Place the banana in the blender. Top up with the milk, seal lid and blend fast for a few seconds until fully liquid.

2. Pour the natural banana shake into a tall glass and dust the top with cinnamon if you like, before drinking.

Apple and Nut Butter

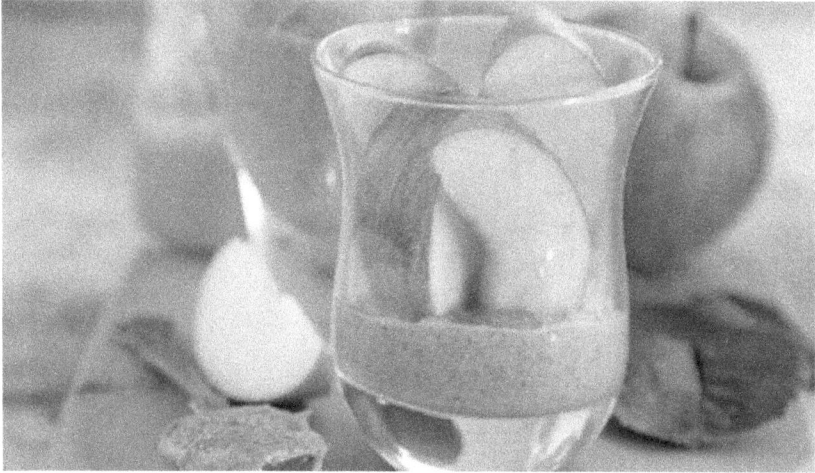

It you are after something earthy, crunchy and different from plain fruit, this combination can make a terrific treat. We know that nut butter is not low fat in large quantities, but here you are only enjoying a small amount.

Why not go for walnut or almond as a healthier alternative to peanut butter – they will still give you some good, healthy omega-3 and omega-6 fatty acids.

Pick a crisp, red or pink apple variety, like Pink Lady for added sweetness and crunch.

Ingredients

- 1 red apple
- 1 tsp of nut butter

Method

1. Slice up the apple into slim wedges and enjoy a dab of nut butter with each slice – so simple, so good.

Finally... 3 Super-Fast, No-Prep Snacks

Here are a few more ideas that take no preparation whatsoever, perfect for your busiest days.

A cereal bar – A great snack for when you are always on the move. Go for a recommended brand from the health food aisle and check that it is not loaded with added sugar, glucose, corn syrup or other calorific sweeteners.

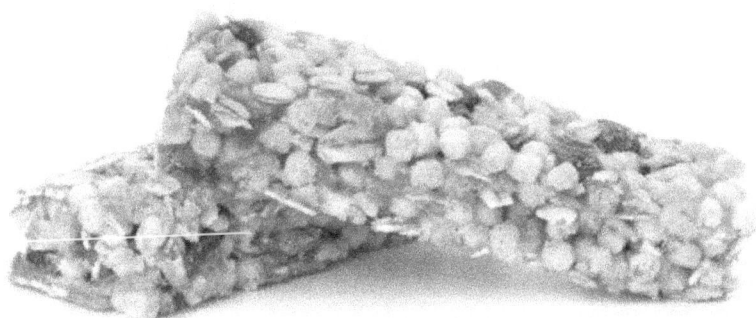

Miso soup – The packets of this savory Japanese broth are available from good health stores and supermarkets. Just empty a sachet into a mug and top up with boiling water. An incredibly low-calorie snack at around 28 calories.

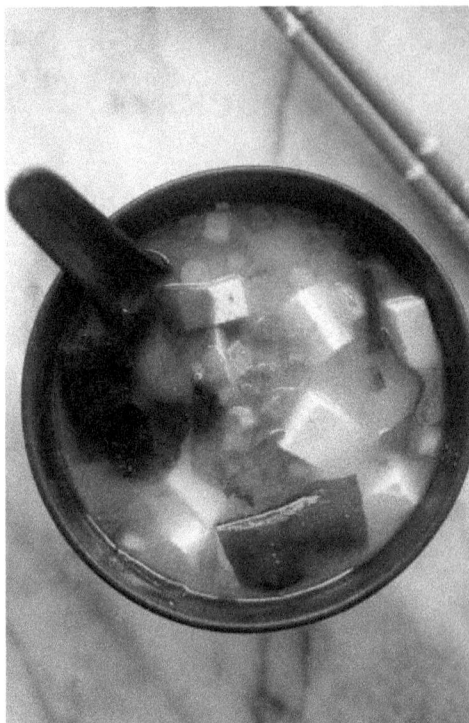

Dark chocolate – Just *three* squares of the best quality stuff you can find, don't get carried away!

Chocolate works wonders for the mood and immunity as it releases feel-good hormone serotonin into the brain and gut. Just what the doctor ordered!

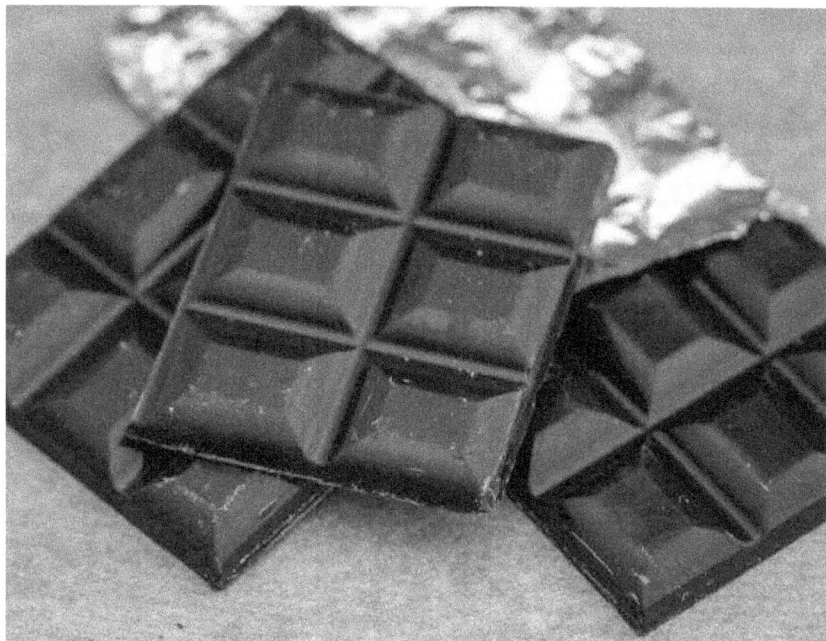

Including these quick options, that makes 14 great, very varied snacks to choose from - 2 per day for your week on the plan.

Mix them up so you don't get bored of the same ones and so that you enjoy more nutrients.

They are fun and good to eat – plus they WILL help you in your quest to lose weight, so enjoy.

Chapter 10

Shopping List

Here's a shopping list with all the ingredients you need for this plan, for your convenience.

The main amounts are mostly stated but not always when it comes to fruit and veg, especially as some people will want to repeat recipes and skip others.

However, we recommend that you only buy the smallest amounts as it is only for 1 week.

Cereal

- Box of unsweetened muesli
- Cereal bars

Milk, dairy and eggs

- Half a pint of semi-skimmed milk
- Natural yogurt
- Reduced-fat cream cheese
- Reduced-fat feta
- Reduced-fat mozzarella
- Reduced-fat goat cheese
- Low-fat yogurt
- Low-fat cottage cheese
- Low-fat crème fraiche
- Low-fat sour cream

- Free-range eggs

Fruit

- Fresh raspberries
- Fresh strawberries
- Oranges
- Plums
- Apples, red
- Bananas
- Lemons
- Limes
- PLUS, fruits portions of your choice

Drinks

- Unsweetened orange juice

Bread Rye crispbreads

- Whole-wheat bagel
- Whole-meal bread, 1 loaf
- Whole-grain crackers
- Whole-wheat pita
- Whole-meal rolls
- Wholegrain tortilla

Vegetables/salad

- Box of cherry tomatoes

- Bag of rocket
- Tomatoes
- Avocado
- Broccoli
- Carrots
- Corn
- Cucumber
- Gem Lettuce
- Green beans
- Kale
- Mushrooms
- Onion
- Large potato for baking
- Radishes
- Red pepper
- Scallions
- Baby spinach
- Sweet potatoes
- Sugar snap peas
- Zucchini
- Oil-free salad dressing

Meat and fish

- 2 lean beef sausages
- 1 chicken breast
- 1 chicken fillet
- 1 cod fillet
- Packet of lean ham
- Packet of king prawns, raw
- Small packet of king prawns, cooked

- 1 lamb chop
- 1 smoked mackerel fillet
- 1 medium salmon fillet
- 1 packet lean turkey breast slices

Tinned or prepared items

- Small tub of low-fat hummus
- Small tin of mixed beans
- Small tin of plum tomatoes
- Small tin of sweetcorn
- Small jar sun-dried tomatoes

Pasta

- Egg noodles

Soups

- Fresh vegetable soup (optional)
- Miso soup sachet

Biscuits and snacks

- Dark chocolate bar
- Cashew nuts
- Nut butter of choice
- Oatcakes
- Popping corn

Herbs, Spices and Store Cupboard Staples

- Arugula
- Balsamic vinegar
- Basil
- Chili peppers, red and green
- Chives
- Cinnamon
- Garlic
- Ginger
- Ground Coriander
- Hot sauce
- Jar of clear honey
- Low-calorie cooking spray
- Olive oil (for cooking)
- Mint
- Mixed dried herbs
- Parsley
- Soy sauce, reduced sodium
- Stock cubes, chicken, vegetable
- Sweet chili sauce, low-calorie
- Thyme
- Turmeric Root
- White wine vinegar
- Wholegrain mustard

If you're enjoying this book and would love to let other potential readers know how great it is, please take a few seconds to leave a review on Amazon.com.

Discover Scientifically-Proven "Shortcuts" & "Hacks" to Lose Weight FASTER (With Very Little Effort)

For this month only, you can get Linda's best-selling & most popular book absolutely free – *Weight Loss Secrets You NEED to Know*.

Get Your FREE Copy Here:

TopFitnessAdvice.com/Bonus

Discover scientifically-proven tips to help you lose weight faster and easier than ever before. With this book, readers were able to improve their weight loss results and fitness levels. So, it's highly recommended that you get this book, especially while it's free!

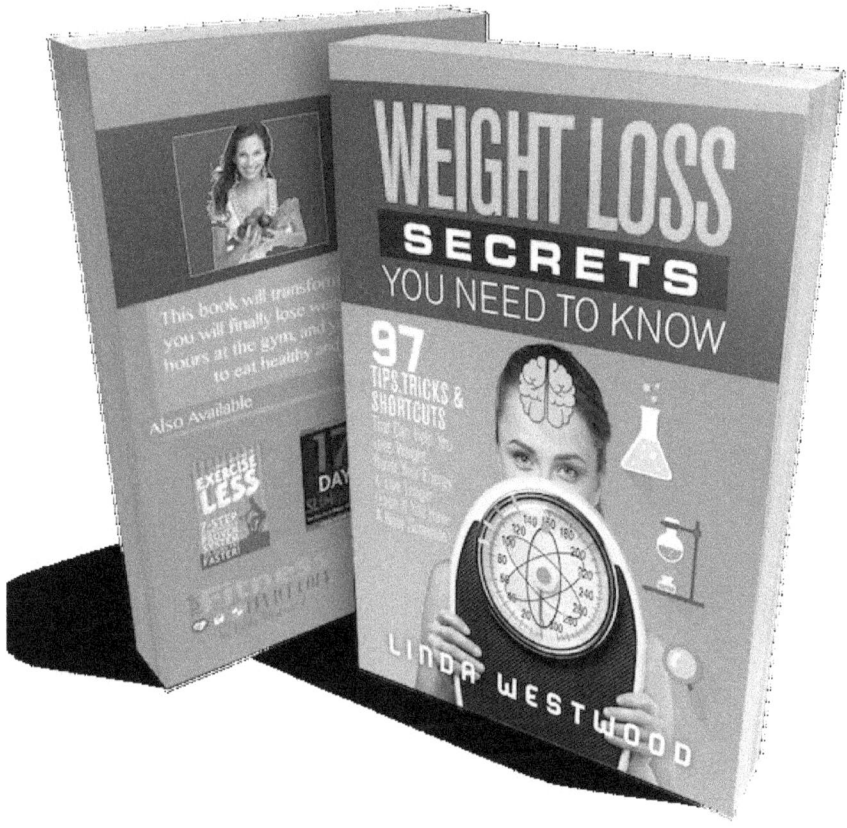

Get Your FREE Copy Here:

TopFitnessAdvice.com/Bonus

Conclusion

Very well done. Your 7 days are over and you are likely you are have undergone a radical change in eating and exercise patterns – time to enjoy the result!

This plan can do so much for your looks and health in just a week.

By following the plan, the majority of people will have boosted your intake of nutrients while lowering your intake of calories, leaving you better nourished than you may have been in a while... but at the same time, much lighter!

Take a look in the mirror now. Chances are you are looking slimmer, with brighter eyes and more glowing skin, especially is you stuck to drinking lots of water throughout the week as advised.

You should congratulate yourself on having achieved considerable internal benefits too – better digestion, fewer toxins in your system, less strain on your joints, heart and organs and a reduced risk of diseases, all of which come with losing weight the healthy way, with exercises included.

You will have speeded up your metabolism, gained in strength and flexibility, and increased tone in your muscles all over, including in the leg, butt and abdomen area...

But most obviously of all, for all of these reasons you will be **looking and feeling great!**

In just 7 days you have effected a transformation inside and out and that is worth celebrating.

Remember:

You stuck to a healthy diet plan and did not starve yourself, eating every 3-4 hours and enjoying snacks.

You carried out a tailor-made exercise plan, without all the usual reps, for toning and smoothing muscles plus burning calories

You have done all you can to accelerate the weight loss process, from drinking water and staying off the alcohol, to sleeping properly and trying detoxifying treats like saunas.

Of course, you know exactly how you need to celebrate it...

Why not go to the wardrobe now and try on that size smaller dress?

You deserve to feel the benefits of your change and it will remind you of how far you have come in a relatively short time.

As dresses may not be as precise every time, you should also measure your inches too and write them down in the dedicated spaces in Chapter 2, just so you can compare them with your 'Before' stats - an exciting moment!

But back to that special dress, if you have one.

If you were always planning to wear it to a party or wedding, or on holiday, we hope you are delighted with the fact that you will look better than ever for the big occasion.

Wear it with pride as you continue to benefit from the low-fat, low-calorie diet and added exercise lifestyle improvements you have made in the past 7 days.

The new habits that you adopted in this plan are changes that, if continued, will ensure your fitness, happiness and health for long into the future.

Enjoying this book?

Check out my other best sellers!

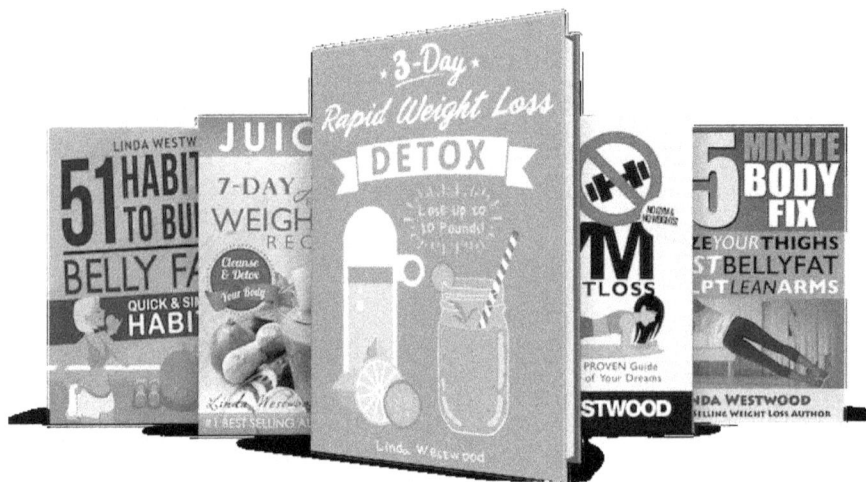

Final Words

I would like to thank you for purchasing my book and I hope I have been able to help you and educate you on something new.

If you have enjoyed this book and would like to share your positive thoughts, could you please take 30 seconds of your time to go back and give me a review on my Amazon book page.

I greatly appreciate seeing these reviews because it helps me share my hard work.

You can leave me a review on Amazon.com.

Again, thank you and I wish you all the best!

www.ingramcontent.com/pod-product-compliance
Lightning Source LLC
Chambersburg PA
CBHW031153020426
42333CB00013B/642